It Took Courage, Compassion, and Curiosity

RECOLLECTIONS AND WRITINGS OF
LEADERS IN CANCER NURSING
1890–1970

Judith (Judi) Bond Johnson, RN, PhD, FAAN
Nurse Consultant
HealthQuest

Susan B. Baird, RN, MPH, MA
Publisher
Meniscus Limited

Laura J. Hilderley, RN, MS
Retired Oncology Clinical Nurse Specialist

Oncology Nursing Society
Pittsburgh, PA

ONS Publishing Division
Publisher: Leonard Mafrica, MBA, CAE
Director, Commercial Publishing: Barbara Sigler, RN, MNEd
Staff Editor: Lisa M. George, BA
Copy Editor: Lori Wilson, BA
Creative Services Assistant: Dany Sjoen

It Took Courage, Compassion, and Curiosity—Recollections and Writings of Leaders in Cancer Nursing: 1890–1970

Library of Congress Card Catalog Number: 2001 088185

ISBN 1-890504-22-X

Publisher's Note
This book is published by the Oncology Nursing Society (ONS). ONS neither represents nor guarantees that the practices described herein will, if followed, ensure safe and effective patient care. The recommendations contained in this manual reflect ONS's judgment regarding the state of general knowledge and practice in the field as of the date of publication. The recommendations may not be appropriate for use in all circumstances. Those who use this book should make their own determinations regarding specific safe and appropriate patient-care practices, taking into account the personnel, equipment, and practices available at the hospital or other facility at which they are located. The editors and publisher cannot be held responsible for any liability incurred as a consequence from the use or application of any of the contents of these guidelines. Figures and tables are used as examples only. They are not meant to be all-inclusive, nor do they represent endorsement of any particular institution by ONS. Mention of specific products and opinions related to those products do not indicate or imply endorsement by ONS.

ONS publications are originally published in English. Permission has been granted by the ONS Board of Directors for foreign translation. (Individual tables and figures that are reprinted or adapted require additional permission from the original source.) However, because translations from English may not always be accurate and precise, ONS disclaims any responsibility for inaccurate translations. Readers relying on precise information should check the original English version.

Printed in the United States of America

Oncology Nursing Society

DEDICATION

On August 27, 1999, the life of a dear friend and oncology nursing colleague came to a premature end. With the death of Patricia "Trish" Greene, RN, PhD, FAAN, at the age of 50, a remarkable woman's chapter in oncology nursing history ended before it could be completed. In her professional lifetime, Trish truly pioneered the care of patients with cancer, while serving as a highly respected role model. She was instrumental in the formation of the Association of Pediatric Oncology Nurses and served as the association's first president. She succeeded Virginia Barckley as a nurse consultant for the American Cancer Society, rising to the position of National Vice President for Patient Services. Her innovative thinking and unending advocacy for quality of life were evident in the many programs for patients and their families that she helped to introduce and guide. At the time of her death, Trish was the Senior Vice President of Patient Services for the Leukemia Society of America, focusing, as always, on quality of life.

Trish's contributions, her potential, and her "chapter" in oncology nursing history were abruptly ended when she died of pancreatic cancer. And so it is with deep respect and great admiration that we dedicate this book to the memory of Trish Greene.

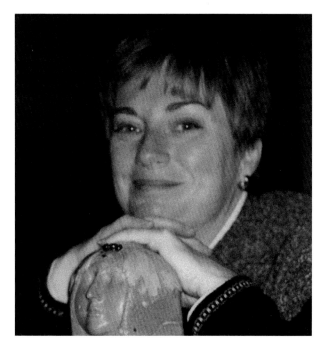

Patricia "Trish" Greene
1949–1999

CONTENTS

FOREWORD

During the last two centuries, nursing emerged as a distinct work assigned the social task of caring for the sick, assisting women in childbirth, and helping the well retain their health. This monumental assignment calls for personal commitment and constant striving for new knowledge and ways to ameliorate human misery. The 12 nurses whose lives are chronicled here offer a luminous view of the varied and real meaning inherent in living a life in modern nursing. With the exception of Rose Hawthorne Lathrop (1851–1926), all did most of their important work in the 20th century. All their stories coincide with the full development and maturing of professional nursing. But they are unique among nurses. They were determined to change the nature of the experience of sickness and thereby, each, in her own way, changed the nature of the practice of nursing.

These women chose to identify with the sickest people they found. People with cancer, a label that attracts fear, despair, and even loathing, drew these nurses on into careers worth remembering. The same forces that created nursing in the first place led these nurses to invent a specialized form of nursing—oncology nursing. They wanted to improve the treatment of the sick by applying their own knowledge and effort, and they wanted to spread new knowledge and technology as broadly as possible. They learned from the people they cared for, each other, and the physicians and other health professionals they knew, and they transformed that knowledge into a new field of understanding and care.

As nurses, they understood people with cancer as strugglers coping with a new personal situation and directed their efforts toward assisting patients with cancer in their crisis. People who do things first have to contend with being different and with the task of explaining and demonstrating their new ideas. Innovators have to reform the professional view of what is right and good in care, and they have to both respond to and direct public opinion toward demanding more and better care. They have to resist the temptation to be parochial and safe in their own environment and go out to teach a better way. In their different lives, these nurses, as you will see, did just that.

They devised ways to help their patients withstand the sometimes devastating effects of chemotherapy, radiation, or surgery. They insisted that people with cancer be treated honestly and without bias. They worked to reveal and confront Americans' avoidance and fear of death. Using every means possible, they raised the standard of knowledge in nursing and taught their students and colleagues to be better nurses.

Scholars are no doubt correct when they say that new specialties emerge because of scientific and technological changes, new ideas of social meliorism, and new patterns of work and professional structure. But I always have been intrigued by the individuals who are the first to step up and

FOREWORD

actually change things. Professions and specialties come into being through the efforts of unusual people who build new types of careers amid changing social and economic circumstances. These women exhibit a kind of wonderful restlessness. As Virginia Barckley said, "you did more than you had to do . . . [it] surpassed any other satisfaction in the world." (p. 89) In one way or another, these 12 all felt compelled to interfere with and change the way people with cancer were being treated. The fruit of their dissatisfaction is a new field of nursing. This is a book about people who helped to lay the foundation for oncology nursing. Oncology nursing—a specialty now about 25 years old—is about organized, systematized learning, research, and care of people with cancer. These 12 lives are a crucial part of its history.

JOAN E. LYNAUGH, MSN, PHD, FAAN

Emeritus Professor and Term Chair
History of Nursing and Health Care
School of Nursing
University of Pennsylvania

PREFACE

Oncology nursing is a young specialty. However, caring for the patient with cancer is not new. As you read about the 12 women highlighted in *It Took Courage, Compassion, and Curiosity—Recollections and Writings of Leaders in Cancer Nursing: 1890–1970*, you will marvel at what they went through just to be able to offer these patients what we today consider standard care. These nursing leaders laid the groundwork for our specialty and the care we provide to our patients every day. You will also see a thread passing through each of these women. Not only does this thread connect each of these leaders, the thread also passes to each of us as cancer nurses and as members of the Oncology Nursing Society (ONS).

Rose Hawthorne Lathrop could be considered a socialite. She was raised with all the comforts of a well-known family. But she recognized the needs of the homeless and poor who were suffering with cancer. What she started in the late 19th century has expanded, and Rosary Hill homes continue to provide care today. Mother Alphonsa, as she later was known, offered hospice care in a time when the word was not even known.

Rosalie Peterson recognized the need for cancer prevention and control. She initially worked for the U.S. Public Health Service and as a public health nurse and later as a consultant who was able to provide education for people about cancer control. As chief of the nursing section of Cancer Control for the National Cancer Institute (NCI), she was in a position to aid in the development of programs for universities and schools of nursing. She worked with other nurses like Katherine Nelson, Doris Diller, and Renilda Hilkemeyer to take the cancer control message to nursing schools and hospitals.

Katherine Nelson was an early advocate for the specialty of cancer nursing. In her role as educator, she was in a key position to advocate for the preparation of nurses to provide care for the patient with cancer. She was an instructor in nursing at the Teachers College at Columbia University and also director of nursing education at Memorial Hospital for Cancer and Allied Diseases. Through this joint position she was able to formulate the first advanced clinical program in cancer nursing, which ran from 1947–1951. She initiated the first course in the United States offering master's and doctoral degrees in clinical specialization. Her efforts led to the role of the clinical specialist of today. Dr. Nelson was an advisor to Lisa Begg, one of the founders of ONS.

Although Edith Wolf did not begin her career in cancer care, she followed in the footsteps of Katherine Nelson at the Memorial Center for Cancer and Allied Diseases as associate director of nursing education. Team nursing and the use of the Kardex System to review patient care were originated by Eleanor Lambertson and introduced to the Cancer Center by Edith Wolf. Patient education was an area of great importance to Edith. Activity with the American Cancer Society (ACS), both on the local and national level, provided Edith with the opportunity to work closely with Virginia Barckley.

Doris Diller began her recognition first as a surgical nurse. She was an instructor without a formal teaching background. Doris appreciated the need for surgical workers to also know the patient. She accompanied all patients on teaching rounds to be sure that their needs were met during this time. Doris was one of the invited faculty members who attended the Institute on Cancer Nursing organized by Rosalie Peterson. As you read through the questions from *A Cancer Knowledge Test for Nurses*, which Doris developed for the Skidmore College Department of Nursing, you can identify common questions of today.

Virginia Barckley's roles as staff nurse, head nurse, visiting nurse, ACS volunteer, National Nurse Consultant for ACS, author, and lecturer have laid much of the foundation of cancer nursing as we know it today. Virginia traveled nationally and internationally in collaboration with members of the ACS National Nursing Advisory Committee to implement innovative programs to improve both skill and knowledge in cancer nursing. Virginia, with Renilda Hilkemeyer, organized the first National Conference on Cancer Nursing in 1973. This conference attracted more than 2,500 participants and was a catalyst that led to the establishment of an organization for nurses in cancer care, now known as ONS.

Renilda Hilkemeyer has represented cancer nursing and cancer nurses during the past 40 years. She began as a consultant in nursing education for the Bureau of Cancer Control for the Missouri Division of Health and was assigned to develop a program to teach healthcare professionals about cancer nursing. This was just the beginning for Renilda. She was appointed as the director of nursing at the M.D. Anderson Hospital and Tumor Institute, a newly opened cancer facility in Houston, TX. She promoted cancer nursing through her involvement with ACS and as a member of the Nursing Advisory Committee. Under the direction of Rosalie Peterson, Renilda served as a consultant to NCI, developing networks and strengthening the visibility of cancer nursing. Renilda's years of dedication to cancer nursing have had an impact on each of us practicing in this specialty today. With Virginia Barckley, Renilda laid much of the groundwork for ONS.

Jo Craytor knew the importance of psychological care of the patient, even while a student nurse. She carried that message to the nursing students in her Fundamentals of Nursing classes at the University of Rochester. To further pave the way for the future, Jo's master's thesis investigated ways that the master's-prepared nurse could be a colleague of the physician. Jo's interest in cancer nursing involved a demonstration project on the team care of patients with cancer. She went on to develop one of the first outpatient chemotherapy clinics at Strong Memorial Hospital in Rochester. Her interest in cancer nursing education continued throughout her career and resulted in the appointment to national advisory committees for ACS and NCI. She holds the distinction of being named the first nurse member of the American Association for Cancer Education.

We all have heard of the hospice movement of the 1970s. This was a time when Dame Cicely Saunders of England lectured extensively about hospice care and St. Christopher's Hospice. As Dean of the School of Nursing at Yale University, Florence Wald was in a position to hear Cicely Saunders. This really sparked her interest in the subject and provided her with the opportunity to not only visit St. Christopher's but also to be instrumental in the development of the first hospice in the United States. As principal investigator of two studies, she was able to provide the evidence of need for hospice services in Connecticut. The Connecticut Hospice of today is based on those pearls that Florence brought back from her stay in London and the results of her research. Florence Wald has served terminally ill patients with cancer in many ways. She and her husband Henry are among the founding members of the International Work Group on Death, Dying, and Bereavement.

Jeanne Benoliel began her career as a nurse researcher and as a cancer nurse following graduate school. This was at a time when cancer nursing was just being recognized but nurses as researchers and scientists were not. This led Jeanne into the world of academia, research, and her doctoral degree. Jeanne realized the need to publish her research and through this began to mentor other nurses who have become leaders in cancer nursing. Jeanne's numerous publications and membership in national and international associations, including ACS, ONS, American Nurses Association, American Academy of Nursing, and the International Workgroup on Death, Dying, and Bereavement, allow us to see the thread continue. Jeanne's recognition as a "Living Legend" by the American Academy of Nursing in 2000 is an honor bestowed on a leader in our field.

Norma Owens entered nursing during the 1950s. Her interest in cancer nursing started, as had others in this book, during a time with the U.S. Public Health Service. Norma began teaching at New York University and worked on both her master's and doctoral degrees. Norma looked at the psychosocial aspects of care, especially those patients undergoing surgery for head and neck cancer that resulted in facial deformity. Norma was involved with both the Sloan-Kettering Institute for Cancer Research and the James Ewing Hospital. During this time, she was instrumental in the beginning of the nursing internship program. This university course offered both professional theory and clinical practicum to provide nurses with the knowledge and skills. Norma was acknowledged for her work with local and regional ACS programs. She also served as a member of the National Advisory Committee of the organization, as have so many of our great leaders.

PREFACE

Louise Lunceford spent most of her cancer-nursing career at the Clinical Center of the National Institutes of Health (NIH). She was faced with clinical trials, adolescents with cancer, and a time when a diagnosis of cancer was not discussed—especially with children. While at NIH, she became involved with the "life island," a new way to protect the immunosuppressed patient. During her time in the education department, Louise had the opportunity to participate in the work-study program sponsored by ACS, allowing her the opportunity to work with Virginia Barckley.

These women all have touched our professional lives. They have been colleagues and friends. Much of what we do today had its foundations in the work of these 12 nurses. We owe them so much. I am honored to have known some of them. Now, through this book, I feel the thread connecting me, you, and ONS to the lives of our nursing leaders.

PEARL MOORE, RN, MN, FAAN
Chief Executive Officer
Oncology Nursing Society

ACKNOWLEDGMENTS

We are indebted to the nursing pioneers whose lives and contributions are chronicled within these pages. They have infused our professional lives, either in person or in the legacies they have left, with the essence of their nursing spirit. Their long and productive lives are models to us and to all who read their stories and writings. We are grateful to the nurses who were able to actively participate in the interview process, to those who took time to relive memories or write tributes, and to family members who helped to enrich the material.

To Joan Lynaugh, the eminent nurse historian who served as advisor and guide to us in the development of this book, we extend our appreciation and admiration. Joan shared her experience and insight into how to establish guidelines and criteria, where to look, and when to recognize that we were ready to write about what we had discovered. Joan helped to light the spark that kept us exploring and building these stories.

To the Oncology Nursing Society (ONS) Board of Directors, we express our appreciation for their receptiveness to the idea of capturing this piece of oncology nursing history. Their recognition of the importance of this project and their support in making it an official project for the ONS Publishing Division is a further example of their wisdom. To the staff, Katina Koontz, archivist, Mark Vrabel, librarian, and Barbara Sigler, Dany Sjoen, and Lori Wilson of the ONS Publishing Division for their help in researching and completing this book.

Finally, we acknowledge the many nurses who were also part of the unfolding of the specialty of oncology nursing during this time period but whose stories are not included here. Quite obviously, there are countless others who made equally important contributions. They too showed courage, compassion, and curiosity. We owe them our lasting respect and offer them our thanks.

THE AUTHORS

INTRODUCTION

A period of accelerated progress in cancer research and treatment began in the early decades of the 20th century, and this progress continues into the 21st century. Surgery emerged as a skilled medical discipline, a rudimentary understanding of x-rays and radium sparked interest in exploring clinical applications, and the complexity of cancer as a category of disease became even more evident. These technological advances required complex postoperative support, with wound and skin care needs frequently exceeding standard care approaches. Areas of care traditionally in the domain of nursing—nutrition, elimination, ventilation, rest, safety, and personal care—posed major challenges when illness was compounded by the side effects of newer cancer treatments.

The professional lives and achievements of 12 women are included in this panorama of cancer nursing pioneers. Their stories become even more meaningful when considered within a series of events in technology and medical management that also contributed to the shaping of nursing practice in cancer care. The process by which care moved from technology to the patient has four steps: identification, diffusion, adoption, and implementation (*Cancer Treatment*, 1988). Consistent with progress in other areas of medical care, technological advances in cancer occurred sporadically, followed by slow and uneven implementation. Each decade reflected some slight change in which new approaches gained acceptability, old ways fell from favor, and different patterns of care eventually emerged. As these professional profiles unfold, readers will find that no clear demarcation exists of precisely when modern cancer care or specialized cancer nursing care began. Although an impressive body of knowledge now constitutes the specialty of cancer nursing, little is actually known about how the patterns of that care emerged; how it was studied, refined and implemented; how it was taught to others through academic, hospital, and continuing-education programs; or how it finally was incorporated into the nursing literature.

Work is one of the ways we define ourselves as we mature; yet work has not been a particular study focus in nursing history. The nursing histories included in this book informally explore what these nurses actually did and how they responded to problems in care and provide the reader with glimpses of how the body of knowledge that currently guides cancer nursing practice evolved.

The primary intent of this book is not to chronicle cancer nursing as a specialty but rather to capture the spirit and contribution of some of its early leaders. It may be helpful for the reader to remember that by 1910, all of the basic components of modern treatment had been identified. The challenges in transferring these advances into clinical practice became readily apparent—physicians needed to develop the skills necessary to deliver and manage the new treatment approaches; hospitals needed to provide appropriately equipped care settings; and nurses needed to meet the care demands accompanying both the disease and its treatment. In addition to providing the com-

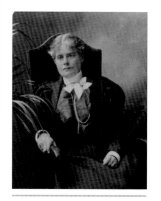

Rose Hawthorne Lathrop

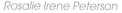

Rosalie Irene Peterson

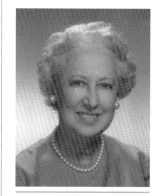

Katherine Nelson

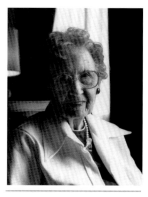

Edith Wolf

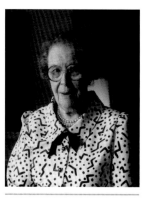

Doris Diller

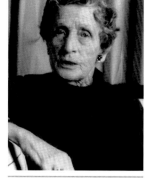

Virginia Barckley

INTRODUCTION

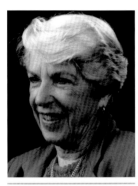

Josephine Craytor

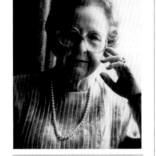

Renilda Hilkemeyer

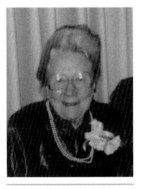

Florence Wald

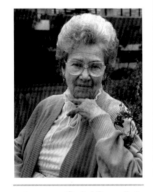

Jeanne Quint Benoliel

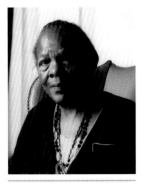

Norma Owens

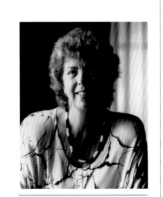

J. Louise Lunceford

fort and caring measures that were already a hallmark of cancer care, trained nurses were called on to manage the care of patients undergoing radical surgery and radiation therapy and, later, those receiving chemotherapy. Persistent and controversial issues complicated care. Whether cancer was hereditary or contagious was uncertain; trained nurses occasionally refused to accept cancer cases because of perceived dangers to themselves ("The Transmission and Care of Cancer," 1907). Recruitment of nurses into the specialty was an ongoing challenge.

New treatments prompted the beginnings of care approaches, constituting a specialized body of nursing care. The stories of the women in this book provide some insight into the beginnings of modern care approaches and how these women, as representatives of many nurses during this time span, helped to develop changes in care. For example, when today's nurse assists the patient recovering from an abdominoperineal resection with peristomal skin care or guides appliance selection and application, a variety of cleansing agents, adhesives, and appliances are available to meet the needs of different situations. Well-defined steps guide the nurse's actions. When British surgeon Ernest Miles introduced this surgery in 1908, such assistive devices did not exist. A rubber-pouch appliance became available in the late 1920s, but disposable appliances were not developed until after World War II.

Wound management alone, without antibiotics and disposable dressing materials, posed tremendous management challenges. William Halstead's radical mastectomy for breast cancer introduced in 1894 (Shimkin, 1979), Wertheim's (1911) extended hysterectomy for gynecologic cancers, and early radiation delivered in doses that were largely uncontrolled, unfractionated, and unshielded posed similar concerns. Many cancer nursing measures that are commonly used today began as responses to these treatments and to the early clinical applications of chemotherapy in the 1940s. The high cancer morbidity and mortality rates that prevailed throughout this period surely prompted the development of nursing approaches to palliation and terminal care.

The stories of the 12 nurses play out against this backdrop. These women came to the settings in which they made their contributions from various backgrounds and educational preparations. Each made individual contributions, but collectively they represent trailblazers in any area of specialization. As authors, we had the good fortune to know almost all of these women personally. We admire them for their willingness to share, then and now.

We applaud the persistent enthusiasm of these women. We readily acknowledge that we could have chosen additional or different nurses to include. As the stories took shape, however, we sensed a mosaic of experience coming together. The book is a collectively robust recollection, a rich past, and a firm foundation.

REFERENCES

Cancer treatment: National Cancer Institute's role in encouraging the use of breakthroughs. (1988, October). Government Accounting Office briefing report to the chairman, Subcommittee on Health and the Environment, Committee on Energy and Commerce, and House of Representatives: Washington, DC.

Miles, W.E. (1908). A method of performing abdominoperineal excision for carcinoma of the rectum and of the terminal portion of the pelvic colon. *Lancet, 2,* 1812–1813.

Shimkin, B. (1979). *Contrary to nature.* Washington, DC: U.S. Department of Health, Education, and Welfare.

The transmission and care of cancer. (1907). *American Journal of Nursing, 8*(3), 200.

Wertheim, E. (1911). *Die erweiternerte abominale operation bei carcinoma coli uteri (auf grand von 500 falen).* Berlin: Urban and Schwartzenberg.

ROSE HAWTHORNE LATHROP
Leader in the Care of People With Incurable Cancer

"I am trying to serve the poor as a servant. I wish to serve the cancerous poor because they are more avoided than any class of sufferers; and I wish to go to them as a poor creature myself . . ."

— *Rose Hawthorne Lathrop*

ROSE HAWTHORNE LATHROP

SIGNIFICANT CAREER CONTRIBUTIONS

- Founder of the Servants of Relief of Incurable Cancer of the Congregation of St. Rose of Lima, Dominican Third Order

- Founded the Dominican Sisters of Charity

- Opened her own cancer hospital, St. Rose's Free Home

RIGHT
Nathaniel and Sophia Hawthorne

Photos courtesy of the Dominican Sisters of Hawthorne

BIOGRAPHICAL INFORMATION

BIRTH AND DEATH

Rose Hawthorne was born on May 20, 1851, in Lenox, MA. She died in her sleep at Rosary Hill in Westchester County, NY, on July 12, l926.

PARENTS

Rose was the third child of Nathaniel Hawthorne and his wife, Sophia. Together with her brother, Julian, and sister, Una, Rose enjoyed a comfortable childhood surrounded by family and many of the most prominent literary, political, and social figures of the time. The Hawthorne family counted as their friends (and some relatives) Ralph Waldo Emerson, Henry David Thoreau, Herman Melville, Robert Browning, Horace Mann, Louisa May Alcott, Oliver Wendell Holmes (the physician), and Henry Wadsworth Longfellow. Rose, Julian, and Una had regular opportunities to be in the company of these notables while the Hawthorne family resided in various Massachusetts communities, including Lenox, Concord, and West Newton. According to one of her biographers, "Rose was a charming, beautiful child, who became a gracious and attractive young girl, who developed into a handsome woman, winning all hearts around her" (Walsh, 1930, p. 30). Her father nicknamed her "Rosebud," a name she carried for many years.

Nathaniel Hawthorne was appointed American Consul to England when Rose was two years old, and the family moved to Liverpool. During their years in England, the Hawthorne children made the acquaintance of many notables such as William Cullen Bryant and Robert and Elizabeth Barrett Browning during dinners in the Hawthorne home. Rose and her siblings always were included at the dinner table, even when their parents entertained such prominent guests.

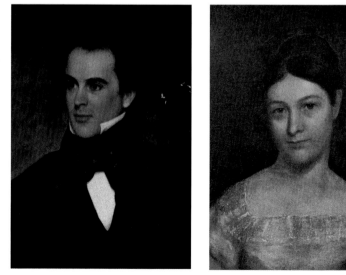

FAMILY

During her early years, formal education was quite erratic for Rose. Julian, Rose, and Una had the best education that could be given to gifted children—an irregular attendance at classes and the constant association with remarkable people. Sophia saw to it that her children were schooled in music and painting, while Nathaniel discouraged his young children's efforts at creative writing. Rose recalled a particular event when she was nine years old. She was retelling a story she had written to a friend, and her father appeared bellowing, "Never let me hear of your writing stories! I forbid you to write them!" (Maynard, 1948, p. 122). Nathaniel considered the female authors of his day a "damned mob of scribbling women" whose novels gave him "no chance of success while the public taste is occupied with their trash" (Valenti, 1991, p. 24).

While living and traveling in Europe, Rose became aware of the art, architecture, and life of the Roman Catholic faith. The Hawthornes were New England Unitarians, and although Nathaniel and Sophia "worshiped" Catholic art, they regarded Catholicism as corrupt. According to Maynard (1948), Catholic life, as witnessed by the observant little Rose in Rome, was not understood in the least, but it had much to do with her later conversion to the Catholic faith.

The Hawthornes returned to Concord when Rose was nine, where she attended formal classes for brief, intermittent periods. She was very close to her father, and in spite of his admonitions to the contrary, Rose continued to dabble in poetry and storytelling.

Nathaniel became depressed over the raging Civil War and the death of his close friend, Thoreau. The Hawthorne family's comfortable lifestyle changed when Rose's father died on May 19, 1864, one day before Rose's 13th birthday. Sophia and her children found themselves in strained financial circumstances. Friends and relatives offered to help with the children's education, which led to the enrollment of Rose in private boarding schools. She took music lessons and continued to paint and write. Rose's church attendance was erratic, and she began to express great boredom with the Unitarian services. Although her conversion to Catholicism was many years away, Rose noted in her memoirs that "in art, Catholicity was utterly bowed to by my relatives and their friends . . . . Glorious scenes were constantly soothing this sense of human sorrow, scenes such as cannot be found in regions outside the Catholic church" (Valenti, 1991, p. 103).

When Rose was 17, her mother decided to sell their home (the Wayside) in Concord and move to Europe. They settled in Dresden where Julian could pursue his engineering studies, Rose could cultivate her artistic interests, and Una's poor health might improve. The Hawthornes became acquainted with the Lathrop family through the American "colony" in Dresden. George Parsons Lathrop was the young man who, according to Sophia, set Rose's "heart beating so fast with his" (Valenti, 1991, p. 42). George returned to New York to attend Law School at Columbia University, and Rose continued her studies in Dresden until war broke out in Germany. She then joined her mother and sister in England in late 1870, and within a few months, Sophia died with a severe respiratory illness.

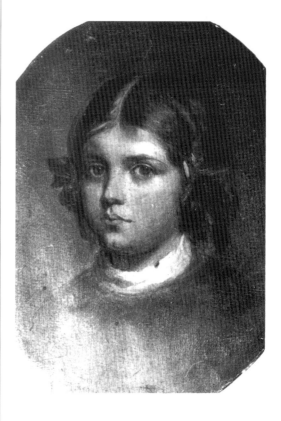

ABOVE
Rose Hawthorne, nicknamed "Rosebud" by her father.

Photo courtesy of the Dominican Sisters of Hawthorne

ROSE HAWTHORNE LATHROP

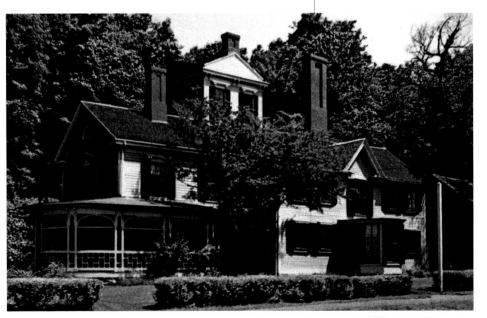

Julian was now head of the family and arranged for the return of his two sisters to America. He sent young George Lathrop to England to accompany Rose and Una on the two-to-three-week ocean journey home. To the surprise of many, Rose and George (both barely 20) announced their wedding plans, and on September 11, 1871, they were married in Chelsea, England, at St. Luke's Anglican Church. George's brother was the only relative from both families in attendance, evidence of the great distress and disapproval of this marriage by the Hawthorne family.

Rose and George sailed for New York to pursue George's new plan to become a writer, having abandoned his thoughts of studying law. Together, he and Rose obtained some of Nathaniel's manuscripts from which to assemble an essay on his last years. Rose was successful in publishing some of her own poetry, and George soon became an associate editor of the *Atlantic Monthly*. Five years after their marriage, Rose became pregnant, and, in addition to the stress over her poor relationship with her brother, she was facing the prospect of pregnancy and childbirth without the support of her mother and sister. A healthy son, Francis Hawthorne Lathrop, was born on November 10, 1876. Rose regained strength, but then "mental distress and hallucinations" began to appear, and she was hospitalized at the McLean Asylum for the Insane. The diagnosis was puerperal insanity, today's equivalent of postpartum psychosis. Rose remained institutionalized for several months, receiving state-of-the-art treatment consisting of warm baths, forced feedings, digitalis to reduce agitation, and opiates to induce sleep.

Although Rose seemed to recover completely from this postpartum illness and was delighted in her son, personal tragedy continued with the death of her sister, from whom she was still estranged. George was in heated disagreement with his editor at the *Atlantic Monthly* and resigned in September 1877, only a few weeks after Una's death. Financially, the Lathrop's were struggling but seemed to be genuinely happy with each other and their son, Francie. George found a position with the *Boston Courier*, and they were able to purchase "The Wayside," which had been Rose's home twice before.

Tragedy struck again when Francie became ill with diphtheria and died within four days on February 6, 1881. Rose and George responded to an invitation from Julian to visit him in England, a gesture of consolation and reconciliation, which they accepted. This was a prelude to the pattern of living apart from each other, which began after the visit with Julian. Rose went to Paris and George to Spain to work on a novel. When they returned to the United States, she went to Concord to sketch and he to Philadelphia to work on another novel. They eventually reunited in New York City, sharing a small apartment and meager incomes from their writing. When Rose inherited a tidy sum from a paternal aunt, she began to plan for separation from George. Rose turned her attention to her circle of women friends in the literary and publishing world, living apart from George for several years. In 1887, George's poor health led both Rose and George to a move from the city, where they lived together in a quiet lifestyle in New London, CT. To the great surprise of family and friends, the Lathrops converted to Catholicism in March 1891. Biographers have speculated about the reasons for such a radical move by two conservative New Englanders. For Rose, Catholicism was perceived as the antithesis of Unitarianism, which was described as "cerebral, excessively rational, unemotional, and masculine" (Valenti, 1991, p. 102). Catholicism to Rose was filled with "tradition, history, humanity, love, and warmth so characteristic of women and so necessary to them" (Valenti, p. 104).

CAREER PATH

One of Rose's dearest friends was the poet Emma Lazarus, whose words are inscribed at the base of the Statue of Liberty. When Emma died a painful death from cancer at the age of 38, Rose was profoundly affected and became acutely aware of the great contrast between the care of affluent patients such as Emma and the abandonment of patients with cancer who were poor. Hospitals had no beds for the destitute with incurable diseases, especially cancer. Most were left to rot and die in damp cellars or wherever they found a space to crawl into. Apathetic authorities sometimes found and moved these destitute people several times before confining them to the almshouse on Blackwell's Island. New York's cancerous poor were warehoused on Blackwell's Island and subjected to horrible conditions. Without proper medical attention or any form of consolation, patients suffered and died.

Rose's fervor and deeper immersion in the Catholic faith gradually led her to question the compatibility of a marital relationship with a life of benevolence and communal existence, which she was exploring. At the age of 44, Rose considered herself a failure at everything she had attempted—art, music, writing, and marriage. She left George and began a retreat at the convent of the Grey Nuns of Montreal, preparing to adopt the life of a nun.

My hope has been to learn nursing, and the way has at last been opened and granted to me. After I have learned this blessed art to some extent and also become familiar with devotional exercises and the care of the souls of the sick and the dying . . . I can intelligently teach the poor, who are ignorant of God, the wonders of his love, [and I wish] to work in New York . . . (Valenti, 1991, p. 128).

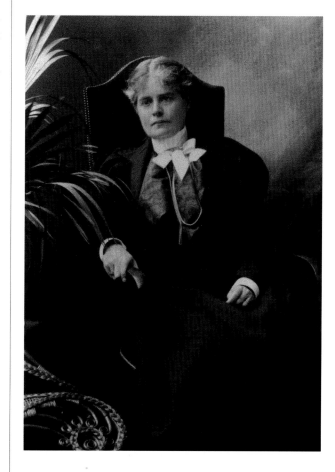

ABOVE
Last formal portrait of Rose Hawthorne Lathrop before she assumed the Dominican habit.

Photo courtesy of the Dominican Sisters of Hawthorne

ROSE HAWTHORNE LATHROP

In 1896, at the age of 45, Rose enrolled in nurse's training at the New York Cancer Hospital (known later as the Memorial Hospital) to learn to care for the dying. She trained for one summer and determined that she knew how to dress the foul, draining lesions as well as tend to the feeding and bathing of the hospitalized patients with cancer. At that time, only those patients whose families could pay for care were hospitalized. The prevailing attitude was that the cancerous poor should not be nursed at all but left to die as quickly as possible. Rose was determined to establish a facility where the cancerous poor could receive the care they deserved. Her plans to open a hospital with six to eight beds on the lower East Side of New York soon changed after searching unsuccessfully for decent space in this squalid section of the city. Whenever she mentioned nursing patients with cancer, potential landlords turned her away. Rose was determined to live and work among the poor in spite of advice from friends and Catholic clergy, from whom she sought support. Maynard (1948) quoted from one of Rose's diaries the following conversation she had with a young priest, from whom she sought help: "My dear Mrs. Lathrop, you are not needed in this locality," he said loftily. "Very little cancer here, I assure you. Besides, the Catholics are moving further uptown, and the Jews are coming in." "Father," Rose returned mildly, "cancer may be far more prevalent than you imagine. Often people have it and are not aware of the fact, and when they are aware of it, they don't always tell everybody. But as for my patients, it doesn't make any difference whether they are Catholics or Jews."

Rose found and rented an abandoned apartment at 1 Scammel Street and proceeded to scrub and paint it marigold yellow, transforming foul, dark space into two reasonable rooms. Nurses at the Henry Street Settlement, from whom she had sought advice on her hospital plans, had encouraged Rose instead to visit patients in their own homes. From her small two-room apartment, Rose began daily excursions into the neighborhood to offer care and support for the cancerous poor in the lower East Side. Word spread quickly, and soon she began receiving the sick in her apartment from 8 am until midmorning, visiting the homebound until 1 pm, then receiving more patients until 5:30 pm. Each evening, she revisited the homebound to apply fresh bandages for the night. Prayer became a regular part of her daily routine, as did observation of the lives of the poor among whom she had settled. Her fear of personal harm disappeared as she was welcomed and even supported in her efforts. Rose invited a few female patients to move in with her and to help her care for others. Mrs.

BELOW
Rose Hawthorne Lathrop
dressing the facial cancer of
Mrs. Watson

*Photo courtesy of the Dominican Sisters of
Hawthorne*

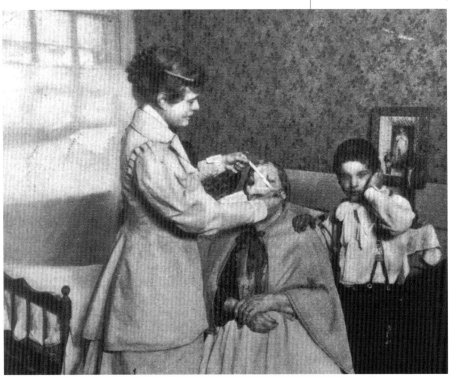

Watson, a woman who had been dismissed from the New York Cancer Hospital when her money ran out, appeared one day seeking attention for her ever-growing facial cancer. Rose remembered Mrs. Watson as being jolly and outgoing (when she had cared for her at the hospital), in spite of being one of the terrible "face cases." Rose invited Mrs. Watson to stay with her and she became a valuable coworker. She saw to it that Rose herself was nursed through a near-fatal bout with pneumonia.

Acquisition of funds to support the work, purchase supplies, and pay the rent was a constant struggle. Rose had used up all of her own money earned from lecturing and speaking engagements prior to this new vocation. Her years as a writer living in literary circles, however, brought continued contact with individuals in a position to help her obtain some financial support. In addition, Rose launched a personal crusade in the form of letters to the editor exhorting the people of New York to contribute to the social and health needs of the poor. She visited prominent and wealthy members of the Catholic faith (not the clergy or Catholic charities) and openly begged for their personal funds to support her work. Rose also visited physicians and other prominent persons of wealth and influence, some of whom became lifelong supporters of the order that she later founded.

Rose became a crusader for the rights of the poor with cancer and for better understanding of cancer as a disease. Cancer was the most dreaded disease of the late 19th century and was believed to be highly contagious. Families, unable to handle the terror of cancer, sometimes expelled their own members to somehow fend for themselves. As part of her drive to prove that cancer was not contagious, Rose not only shared her living quarters but also supplies, food, and kitchen utensils with her patients. She did believe in absolute cleanliness and hand washing, but later, when rubber gloves became available, she forbade their use because of the message that might be conveyed to patients with cancer. Rose believed that using rubber gloves to cleanse and dress patients and their lesions would interfere with patients' feeling of acceptance by the caregiver.

In March 1897, Rose was forced to find new quarters for her clinic when the condemned Scammel Street building was torn down. This time, she managed to find space in a Water Street building with four rooms on each of the two floors. The rooms and beds immediately were filled with patients with cancer, and Rose felt that she at last had her hospital. In spite of the crowding and shared space, every effort was made to preserve dignity by screening patients during dressing changes. Curious friends came to see what Rose was doing, and when a few volunteered their time, she assigned them to read or just sit and chat with the patients. She believed that pleasant surroundings and diversions for the mind were essential to easing the burden of incurable cancer.

Rose actively recruited trained nurses but rejected as many as she kept because she judged their motivation or behavior to be inappropriate. None of the nurses were paid for their services. Some

"A fire was then lighted in my heart, where it still burns . . . I set my whole being to bring consolation to the cancerous poor."

ROSE HAWTHORNE LATHROP
(MAYNARD, 1948, P. 2)

ROSE HAWTHORNE LATHROP

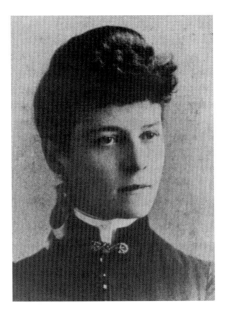

ABOVE
Alice Huber made a lifelong commitment to join Rose in nursing the cancerous poor.

Photo courtesy of the Dominican Sisters of Hawthorne

of the occasional volunteers became full-time caregivers, overcoming their initial revulsion at the sights and constant odors.

Rose's deep belief in the need for and importance of nursing those with cancer is underscored in a letter written to Sister Marie Elise of Mount St. Vincent's-on-the-Hudson. Sister Marie Elise had sent a young woman to help at the Water Street house, to which Rose replied, "Send me more strong young women or delicate brave ones! No better life, I am more and more convinced, can be carried on by women of intelligence, and I long to have truly intelligent and noble women adopt it, for I can never myself make it the growth it should be" (Maynard, 1948).

Alice Huber entered Rose's life and work in December 1897. Alice was a painter and an art instructor in New York who was sent to see Rose after consulting with Father Fidelis of the Cross about her desire to find "spiritual perfection." Alice had read newspaper accounts of Rose's work with the cancerous poor and wanted to meet her. Alice, like so many others, was unprepared for the poor and bare facility and the malodorous atmosphere. In spite of her initial feelings of revulsion and horror at what she encountered, something about Rose caused Alice to stay and volunteer for a few afternoons per week. The affinity between these two women grew quickly, and, in March 1898, Alice joined Rose in a lifelong commitment to nursing the cancerous poor.

George Lathrop had continued his work in the literary world after Rose left him to pursue nursing. He was modestly successful with the opera he had made of Hawthorne's *The Scarlet Letter* but totally unsuccessful in his attempts to win Rose's return. In April 1898, George died from cirrhosis of the liver before Rose was able to reach his bedside. Although she was the one who had walked away from their marriage, Rose always had hoped that George someday would understand her work and join her in it. With the death of her husband, Rose felt freed from the marriage bond and took steps toward functioning under the auspices of traditional Roman Catholic religious practices. She and Alice cut their hair, donned garments similar to a habit, and sought permission from the Archbishop of the Diocese of New York, Michael Augustine Corrigan, to form a nursing order. Although the Bishop did allow the women to continue wearing the habit of a nun, he refused their request to establish an order or to allow them to work under ecclesiastical supervision.

Rose never had given up on her dream to open a true cancer hospital, and with the $9,500 she had managed to accumulate through her steady pleas, she purchased property on Cherry Street, naming it St. Rose's Free Home. The name was selected not because of her own but in a random drawing from the names of saints that she and Alice had written on slips of paper. Rose was criticized in the press for not working in an established hospital, but this home, with beds for 20 women, was precisely the setting she wanted. She was convinced that doctors were not needed to care for those without hope of recovery, and she also believed that the hospitalized terminally ill were often subjects of experimental surgery. Rose spoke openly about the "institutionalized neglect of cancer patients . . . where feelings of courteous pity and earnestness among doctors and nurses was lacking." She also believed that (hospital) "administrators commanded high salaries, but practiced false economy with regard to needs of their charges" (Valenti, 1991, p. 165).

A young Dominican priest, Father Thuente of St. Vincent's, came to thank Rose and Alice for the care they were providing for one of his parishioners. He became aware of their deep desire to become members of an order and quietly intervened on their behalf with the bishop. Under Father Thuente's instructions, Rose, Alice, and Cecilia Higley were accepted as secular tertiaries living in the world. In September 1899, Rose founded the specialized group of tertiaries, The Servants of Relief of Incurable Cancer of the Congregation of St. Rose of Lima, which forms part of the Dominican third order. Rose took the name of Sister Mary Alphonsa, Alice became Sister Mary Rose, and Cecilia became Sister Mary Magdalen. These names, however, could not be used except in private.

The work of Rose and Alice did not go unnoticed, in part, because of Rose's persistence in fund-raising through letters and articles in the New York newspapers and her constant requests to friends and acquaintances for financial contributions. Rose included detailed descriptions of individual patients and their struggles as part of her plea. She was not against shaming her friends in their comfortable lives, and they responded with small, but steady, contributions. Rose was not in favor of fund-raising from teas or social events, refusing to accept money raised in this manner. She believed that charity should be supported by individual, personal gifts.

Archbishop Corrigan was well aware of the work of The Servants of Relief of Incurable Cancer, and, after a year of what he described as "an extremely rigorous novitiate," he instructed Father Thuente to give

CONSTITUTIONS OF THE SISTERS OF RELIEF

Among the provisions in the constitution of the Sisters of Relief are the following
(from Maynard, 1948, pp. 368–369):

- Only the very poor who are suffering from cancer in its last stages are to be received.
- Those received shall always be treated with the utmost consideration.
- There is to be no harsh speaking to any patient, and no shrinking from close contact.
- There are to be no experiments with the patients, no use of knife or even of radium is allowed.
- No paid nurses are to be employed, except a male orderly for the men.

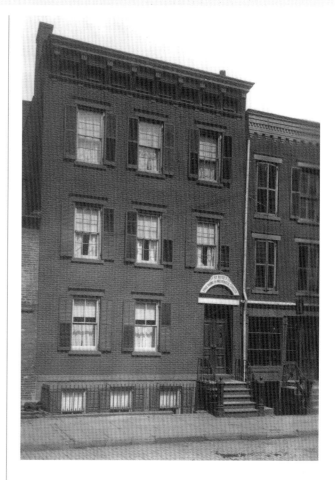

ABOVE
St. Rose's Free Home
426 Cherry Street
New York
1899

Photo courtesy of the Dominican Sisters of Hawthorne

ROSE HAWTHORNE LATHROP

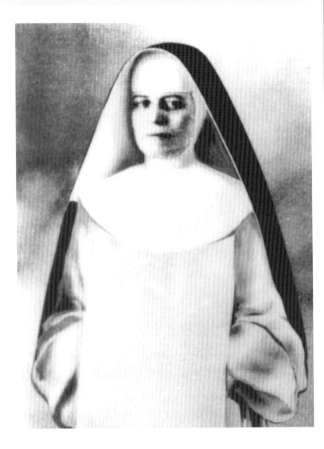

ABOVE
Sister Mary Rose (Alice Huber)

Photo courtesy of the Dominican Sisters of Hawthorne

the secular tertiaries the Dominican habit. On December 8, 1900, the sisters made their final vows and officially were known as Sister Alphonsa, Sister Rose, and Sister Mary.

Sister Alphonsa had struggled for a number of years with the awareness that men needed care for their cancers as much as women did. However, not enough space or help was available to allow men to be admitted to the Cherry Street house, and the sisters had to content themselves with dressing the men's cancers in the relief room where people came to seek rent money, used clothing, and groceries. The relief room also served as a type of outpatient clinic where the sisters treated other illnesses in addition to cancer.

Moved by the plight of a destitute former British military officer with advanced cancer, Sister Alphonsa managed to rent a few rooms across the street to accommodate her first male patient. The Annex, as it was called, was hardly satisfactory, as the sisters had to rely on the janitor to look after the few male patients at night. The drunken janitor often would fail to keep the furnace going, and, during winter months, the patients suffered as much from the freezing cold as from their cancer. Sister Alphonsa set her sights on finding much larger quarters that would accommodate patients of both sexes. She began a novena to the Sacred Heart, enlisting the other sisters, patients and their relatives, and her many friends to join in the effort. As if in answer to their prayers, Sister Alphonsa was visited by a priest from a French Dominican order, who offered to sell her its large home in Westchester County, NY. The sisters, knowing they did not have money for a purchase, set out by train to see for themselves this home near the village of Sherman Park. As they approached the grounds, they were overwhelmed by the beautiful country setting on a hill surrounded by trees, gardens, a grape arbor, and greenhouses filled with flowers. The house had 60 rooms and a porch that ran the circumference of the building. The Dominican fathers sold this magnificent nine-acre property to the sisters for $28,000, accepting a down payment of $1,000, which was all that the sisters could afford. In June 1901, The Servants of Relief of Incurable Cancer took over the property, naming it Rosary Hill Home, and prepared to make it habitable for their patients. Sister Alphonsa was to be the superior general for Rosary Hill and the Cherry Street Homes in New York City, and, as such, became known as Mother Alphonsa. She and a group of postulants tackled the thankless task of cleaning and supervising renovations, finding themselves exhausted from working and covering the distance within the huge building. The renovations reflected any new homeowner's worst nightmares, as they dealt with contaminated groundwater from leaking oil drums and an inadequate heating system during the winter. Constant strong winds on the hilltop location slammed doors, tore at open windows, and could unbalance a person standing on the porch. Sudden rainstorms meant wet floors, because no one could move the distance through the building quickly enough to close all of the windows. In spite of it all, no one could deny the clear advantages of being away from the hot, crowded city, and Rosary Hill soon filled with male and female patients from the slums of New York City.

Mother Alphonsa never despaired over any of the structural problems or the constant need for money. She knew that her patients were experiencing a contentment they had never known before. She encouraged them to be outside walking in the woods, puttering in the greenhouses, or just resting on the great porch. Mother Alphonsa believed that this peaceful setting sometimes added months to patients' lives.

With the opening of Rosary Hill in 1901, Mother Alphonsa began publication of a monthly news magazine, *Christ's Poor*. She referred to this publication as a "monthly report" and wrote most of it herself. The content of *Christ's Poor* focused on the caring activities of the sisters, listing their needs and those of their patients, along with a financial statement. Names of donors were published regularly, and specific patients were profiled. For the entire duration of its publication (1901–1904), Mother Alphonsa included statements about her philosophy of charitable giving in the column "The Objects of the Work." She believed that the public was willing and able to provide for her charitable work, as evidenced by the fact that she never solicited or received state aid or funds from Catholic charities.

Mother Alphonsa took an active role in the training of novitiates as well as in patient care and in the management of Rosary Hill. She lectured the sisters with her beliefs in their role and in the philosophy of the order as set down in the constitutions of the Sisters of Relief.

Now that male patients could be accommodated in the large quarters at Rosary Hill, Mother Alphonsa observed that the men seemed to rebound very quickly from a pale, weak, and bedridden state to one of wanting to help. Although their prognosis was unchanged, the male patients gladly volunteered to move furniture and work in the gardens. Mother Alphonsa believed that the sheer beauty of the surroundings at Rosary Hill did much to lift the spirits of all patients, particularly the men who gathered regularly on the porches to talk, read papers, and smoke. (Smoking was forbidden inside the large wooden structure.) Patients were allowed great freedom to do as they pleased, even if it meant staying in bed all day or retiring early for the night.

Mother Alphonsa had long nourished the hope that men could be induced to enter the nursing field specifically to care for male patients. Rosary Hill could afford only one orderly, and a steady turnover occurred in their services. At one point, Mother Alphonsa tried to convince Brother Dutton (a Trappist Monk working among the lepers in Molakai) to establish a charity for male patients with cancer, similar to the Servants of Relief. She had hoped that Brother Dutton would gather men who did not feel they were called to the priesthood but were willing to give their lives to God in tending to the sick. Although Brother Dutton declined the invitation because of advanc-

"The report of the financial state of our humble Homes is not reassuring, except that we can say we have always escaped disaster, and expect to do so now."

Payments made in September for Rosary Hill Home

Feed for livestock	38.30
Plumbing and boiler setting	36.70
Bread, expressage, and stamps at village depot	45.26
Clothing	7.10
Carpentry	15.38
Drugs	20.68
Man on farm	5.00
Engineer and general worker	55.00
Barber for male patients	2.75
Total	226.17

Amount spent in St. Rose's Home, Cherry Street, for September

Groceries, fruit, and vegetables	31.27
Meat bill	22.80
Bread bill	4.60
Rolls and cake	2.80
Small sundries	14.30
Woman to help	7.40
Total	83.17

(MAYNARD, 1948, PP. 361–362)

ROSE HAWTHORNE LATHROP

ing age and his devotion to the leper colony, Mother Alphonsa did not give up praying that he would change his mind.

The quest for more and better facilities continued. Donations were sought to purchase and renovate a large home in New York City, replacing the Cherry Street Home. The new St. Rose's Home was opened in 1912. Meanwhile, Rosary Hill proved to be fairly costly to operate because of its age, construction, and inefficient heating system. An even greater concern was the threat of fire in this wooden, windswept building. In her usual style, Mother Alphonsa selected a site near Rosary Hill, began planning the new structure, and launched one of her more vigorous fund-raising campaigns. At the same time, she increased her efforts to recruit greater numbers into the order, insisting that paid nurses would not work in any of the sister's homes. The policy of accepting only those patients who were penniless also was continued.

By the spring of 1926, Mother Alphonsa had raised more than half of the $317,000 projected for construction of the new home. She continued her practice of sending handwritten thank you notes to every donor, even those whose gifts amounted to a few dollars. At the age of 75, she saw the beginning of the construction on the new home that she had helped to design, ensuring that sunshine entered every room for at least part of the day. Mother Alphonsa believed that compassionate

BELOW
Rosary Hill Home
Hawthorne, New York

Photo courtesy of the Dominican Sisters of Hawthorne

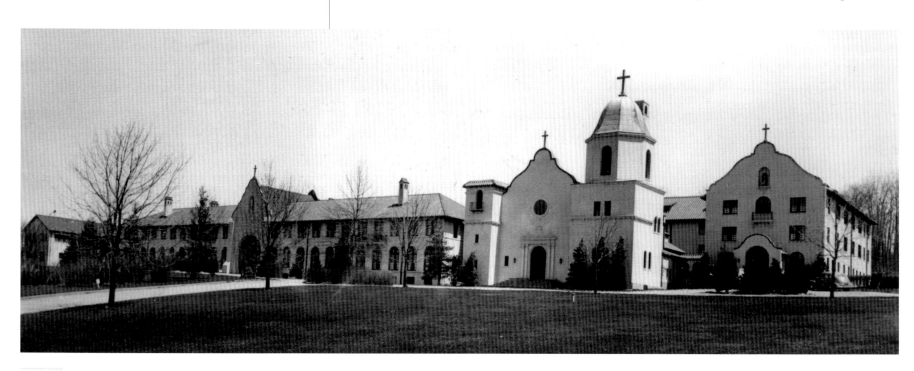

care and bright, pleasant surroundings did more for the relief of both body and soul of the cancerous poor than any medical treatment. This belief was upheld in the new home at Rosary Hill, which she did not live to see to completion. Mother Alphonsa died in her sleep at Rosary Hill on July 12, l926.

SUMMARY

Mother Alphonsa's legacy of nursing care for impoverished patients with cancer continues today in the seven homes owned and operated by the Dominican Sisters of Hawthorne, NY. In addition to those in Hawthorne and in New York City, homes are located in Atlanta, GA, Cleveland, OH, Fall River, MA, Philadelphia, PA, and St. Paul, MN.

Many of the principles of cancer care that Mother Alphonsa espoused in the late 19th and early 20th centuries are still valid today. Simply stated, she believed in and promoted the following:

- Nondiscrimination on the basis of age, sex, race, or religious preference.
- Cancer is not contagious.
- Males are capable and willing providers of nursing care.
- Clean, bright surroundings and fresh air help to ease suffering from cancer.
- Companionship and reasonable activity are important, even for the terminally ill.
- Financial support for the destitute patient with cancer can be sought and obtained from the public at large.
- Selfless, dedicated individuals can and will provide uncompensated nursing care for the poor who are terminally ill.

REFERENCES

Burton, K. (1937). *Sorrow built a bridge*: *A daughter of Hawthorne*. London: Longmans, Green and Company.
Code, J.B. (1929). *Great American foundresses*. New York: MacMillan Company.
Maynard, T. (1948). *A fire was lighted*. Milwaukee, WI: Bruce Publishing Company.
McKown, R. (1966). *Heroic nurses*. New York: G.P. Putnam's Sons.
Valenti, P.D. (1991). *To myself a stranger. A biography of Rose Hawthorne Lathrop*. Baton Rouge, LA: Louisiana State University Press.
Walsh, J.D. (1930). *Mother Alphonsa, Rose Hawthorne Lathrop*. New York: MacMillan Company.

"There is a rather fantastic estimate in the world about the sacrifices that nurses of the cancerous poor must make. And certainly there is an element of courage in befriending the kind of people we befriend. But everybody who lives a vigorous kind of life has to exercise courage even to live . . . unless one is a lizard! . . . The time may come when, with the discovery of a cure for cancer, this work of ours will become a fossil. But we haven't got there yet. Our function in the world is to do something for the terrible sorrow those know to whom no pity is given."

MOTHER ALPHONSA
(MAYNARD, 1948, P. 367)

ROSE HAWTHORNE LATHROP

SELECTED WRITINGS

FROM THE DIARY OF ROSE HAWTHORNE LATHROP

I took a streetcar anxiously one day, a Sunday, in order to hunt for the region in the city which should strike me as best fitted for my attempt at nursing among the poor. I prayed to Our Lord to give me intelligence to know when I had come to the place He willed me to settle in, if He so willed. The East Side proved much the most crowded and desperate.

As soon as I could take another afternoon from my Hospital work, I wandered about the East Side, looking for the very street and the sort of house where I should conclude to make inquiries. It was a lonely and frightened season in my determination; but I always thrust the care upon Our Lord, assuring Him that I knew my incapacity. I was alarmed by the faces I saw, both of men and women, and feared that I should be robbed and even murdered, if I lived alone among such characters. As I found my announcement of desiring to bring cancer patients into the apartments about which I negotiated, made everyone draw back in dismay, I concluded to appeal to a real estate agent.

The real estate agent was deeply interested at once, as he had lost his father by cancer six weeks before. He elaborately described his father's illness, and his own nursing of him, and assured me that he would do all in his power to find me a small house, or an apartment.

As he sent me no further word, in a day or two I called upon him again, and got the address of a house on Scammel St., corner of Henry St. Every window pane was broken, the house seemed abandoned, and a defunct liquor store formed the base of the broken-down abode; but it was just what I should have liked to take, if I had the money to repair it a little, and if the whole block had not just been bought by the city for a school building. Feeling very brave, and crossing myself, I opened the door in the wooden fence of the yard, and, after greeting a cat with a green and a blue eye, set out to look through the house; making up my mind to it by realizing that if I turned away in dread, my cowardice would upset all my future efforts, where similar alarms would most likely be numerous.

Instead of concealed thieves and cutthroats, I found a good-natured Irish family stowed silently away upstairs. A fierce dog in the basement would, however, have closed my earthly career, they said, if I had stumbled upon him first. The family revealed the short lease of existence of the building, and so I had to put aside all desire for it. I began to be heavy of heart at the difficulties in hiring a place in which to begin my work; and I allowed myself to wonder whether God intended at last to show me that my work was not in this field.

It became so discouraging to look for rooms that I decided to appeal to the priest of the Church nearest to the quarter I had selected for my search; and I found a young priest at St. Mary's one morning. He set out to annihilate me, by manner and speech, probably thinking me a perfect fool. He said: there was very little cancer hereabouts; that the Catholics were all moving uptown, and the Jews moving into this neighborhood; and he gazed his contempt over my shoulder.

I answered that cancer was very prevalent, though not often known even by those afflicted with it; that it made no difference whether my patients were Catholics or Jews; and that I hoped, if I came into the parish, he would give me advice.

I had been told that there was a nice apartment on Scammel St. and I reluctantly concluded to hunt that up first; yet was convinced it would be too expensive, and moreover, not the kind of quarters I wished to occupy, as I wanted to be of the poor as well as among them. A prominent little sign of "Floor to Let" at No. 1 Scammel St. caught my eyes; and penetrating darkness and dirt and shattered stairs, I looked at the empty rooms, all unlocked and forlorn, two little cells being almost entirely shut off from air and light by a house-wall close to the windows, and I immediately decided to take this apartment. In every respect it answered my idea; it was as inconvenient, as devoid of necessary arrangements as any poor person could have endured; and, on the other hand, there was an absence of liquor saloons.

. . . Near the house trip along unceasing cars all day and night, and a pleasant little square gives breathing space; and between the houses, across the way, the moon makes glorious scenes of cloud and light, while the salt breezes drift over pretty freshly from the harbor. The black holes which I had looked upon as hideous bedrooms are gladdened in the mornings by a miraculous sunbeam, shooting in at a little square window high up in one chamber-wall, and rays that insist upon coursing across the little sitting-room through the doorway of the second sleeping-apartment.

The frightful dirt everywhere was scrubbed and painted into flight, and light colors have sent thrills of ecstasy through every bosom that has felt relief from the sorrowful tints existing before in this tenement. Smells have vanished also, and the very crannies which were most repulsive have, by special attention, become almost fascinating.

The Jewish woman on the ground-floor, who was called "that thing" by the other tenants, shines with happy smiles now, and everybody is growing to love her, because I like her, and said respectfully that she had a soul, and Our Lord loved her, and she was very kind indeed to me.

The lady over me who was said to be unbearable, because she fought so unmercifully with her husband, has been so good to me that I have wept a little over her thoughtfulness, her tea, and her gentle accents.

———

I went to the Board of Health to ask if I should be permitted to nurse patients without the constant supervision of a doctor, and learned that there was no hindrance. The functionary whom I saw was arrested by the word "cancer," and told me that his wife had died of the disease. It is impressive to find how often people have this seldom-mentioned disease at the very core of their history; and a silence occurs before they reveal particulars to me which I have come to understand is the prelude to revelations. The interest these people take in my undertaking satisfies even me. First comes the tremulous question: "Have you found that cancer can ever be cured?" Then they cannot talk enough of the great sorrow, or dread of a recurrence in the case of a child who seems to be cured, and so on.

The interest, the incentives which invigorate every day of a nurse who works with love, is to perceive the hungry longing of patients, and those who love them, for sympathy and relief. The flattery of being needed so much is sweet as any there is . . . .

The repulsion once overcome, one wonders that there was any hesitation in deciding to eradicate so dreadful a state of affairs. So in deciding to listen to the moaning appeal of a sufferer, or to attend to the loathsome state she is in, we suddenly find ourselves afire with enthusiasm, because without us this sufferer would have been without love—without relief: Horrible thought! Let those who desire to keep the fire of charity from their hearts, never come near the agony of the poor.

Note. From *Rose Hawthorne Lathrop, Selected Writings* (pp. 138–142) by D. Culbertson, 1993, Mahwah, NJ: Paulist Press. Copyright 1993 by D. Culbertson. Excerpted with permission.

TRIBUTES

Rose Hawthorne (Mother Alphonsa) devoted her life to compassion for others. The Hawthorne Dominican Sisters and staff members at the seven homes have carried on her service, affording consolation to patients and their families as well as influencing and enriching the lives of countless volunteers. These effects are profound and lasting. An example of such influence is evident at Our Lady of Good Counsel Home in St. Paul, MN. My late husband, Dr. LeRoy Geis, began volunteering at the home in the mid-1960s. Our children often would accompany him on rounds. Sister Patrick (one of Dr. Geis' closest confidants and mentor in the order) gave our children snacks, serving the dual purpose of entertaining and occupying the children while Dr. Geis attended to business. Dr. Geis continued to serve the patients, their relatives, and the sisters until his death on St. Patrick's Day in 1995. He always said that, "The home is the closest place to heaven on earth."

Because our children were nurtured and influenced by the sisters, almost since birth, they enjoyed being at the home. It was their idea during Lent years ago to serve the patients their Sunday noon meal. Our youngest son, Brian, was too small to feed the patients, so he visited and assisted with the dishes. This practice continues today and now includes every Sunday and each of the holidays. Serving the patients (guests of the home) and their relatives is a joy, whether in their beautifully decorated rooms or in the lounge. In addition to our immediate family (including two granddaughters), we have enlisted friends who, like us, know helping the sisters is a privilege. In this day and age, finding serenity and tranquility amid our chaotic lives is difficult. However, being in the home gives one a feeling of being at peace and closer to God. In addition, there is solace (inexplicably received) that we are able to carry with us until and especially at our end.

Lives of our family members have been made much richer and fuller by working with the followers of Mother Alphonsa. The sisters' happiness, seen in their smiles and actions, fills the home. They have been role models for the past 35 years for each life they have touched, including our five grown children, their spouses, and two granddaughters. We have become comfortable among the terminally ill and their relatives. Our children have grown to be compassionate and empathetic toward others both in and out of the home, as evidenced by their choice of service professions: a mother, farmer, doctor, and teacher. Volunteering is part of their everyday living. Our youngest son, for example, in addition to completing his studies, takes care of his mother and a 93-year-old neighbor. Rose Hawthorne's influence of devotion and compassion will live on through the LeRoy Geis family and countless others.

Dorothy P. Geis, RN, BSN, MEd

St. Paul, MN

ABOVE
Mother Alphonsa (Rose Hawthorne Lathrop)

Photo courtesy of the Dominican Sisters of Hawthorne

ROSE HAWTHORNE LATHROP

Our homes are far from full of sorrow. To say nothing of the happiness of the Sisters, who are profoundly interested in succoring these poor, and have a life which is as much of heaven as they will accept, the patients are almost always as contented as are people in the active world. The cancer patients adapt ideas to their state, and every, little thing helps to brighten it. Some read a great deal, especially the men; and some women sew a great deal. In both departments, the ornamental months of the year are largely spent in gazing at things from the piazzas and summerhouses, the men with their pipes and the women with their tongues. There are plenty of pet birds of various kinds, and there are fishes and newspapers and music in daily swirl of attractiveness, much enhanced by the pet dogs, but not more startling than the feline jousts. Some patients live for a number of years, against all prophecies, becoming very dear friends to the Sisters. It seems as if in no section of human existence could persons be more admirable, on an average, than cancer patients as the Sisters see them, indeed it seems as if no class held such, brave, devout nonsense-free human beings. (Excerpt: "Two Homes That Smile as One," Mother M. Alphonsa Lathrop, 1926)

During the last year of her life, Mother Alphonsa wrote the short essay titled "Two Homes That Smile as One." She saw the embodiment of her dream coming to life within the community of Sisters she founded working in the two homes she established, St. Rose's Home and Rosary Hill Home. Her homes still in existence are now seven and remain dedicated to her principles of amelioration of life for the poor suffering with incurable cancer through the provisions of loving home-like dwellings and dedicated nursing Sisters who strive to promote comfort and relieve pain. Mother Alphonsa once said, "If our Lord knocked at the door, we should not be ashamed to show what we have done." Today her words and her charisma seem just as real and alive in the Sisters who live her ideals. Although the homes now have solariums and sun parlors to replace the summer houses and a few of the men smoke pipes, a walk through any of the homes of the Dominican Sisters of Hawthorne gives evidence of Mother Alphonsa's legacy: her great service to the poor with incurable cancer in her work of more than 100 years.

Sister Mary de Paul, OP

Director of Nursing
Rosary Hill Home
Hawthorne, NY

Professional papers and effects of Rose Hawthorne Lathrop are located in the archives at Rosary Hill Home in Hawthorne, NY; Houghton Library, Harvard University, Cambridge, MA; Talbot Collection, Georgetown University, Washington, DC; and the Manuscript Division of the New York Public Library (Century Collection and Albert A. Berg Collection).

ROSALIE IRENE PETERSON, MSN, RN
Leader in Cancer Education—Prevention and Early Detection

"For a really effective cancer control program, the nurse must contribute more than expert bedside nursing care. She must be on the alert to recognize precancerous and early cancer signs. Case finding, often regarded as a function of the public health nurse, is also a responsibility of the hospital nurse."

— Rosalie Irene Peterson

ROSALIE IRENE PETERSON

SIGNIFICANT CAREER CONTRIBUTIONS

- Created and delivered cancer control programs on American Indian reservations

- Coordinated the Cancer Control Program of the U.S. Public Health Service

- Directed the writing of a book that incorporated information on cancer throughout nurses' basic educational program

- Project Director of the first program that awarded federal grants to schools of nursing to improve cancer nursing for students who were training at the basic level

RIGHT
Peterson Family
Rosalie (front right), father,
Gustavus (front left), mother,
Ida, and brother, Ralph

BIOGRAPHICAL INFORMATION

BIRTH AND DEATH

Rosalie Irene Peterson was born June 19, 1900, in Lindsborg, KS, and died July 8, 1985, in Peoria, AZ.

PARENTS

Rosalie was one of two children born to Gustavus Gottfried Peterson and Ida Agusta Young. Rosalie's parents immigrated to America from Sweden. Gustavus was the second oldest of 12 children. Most of his siblings also immigrated to America. He and his wife chose to settle first in Minneapolis, MN, where his older brother was living. Their first child, Ralph Arthur, was born in Minneapolis in 1897. The family moved to Lindsborg while Ralph was still an infant; Rosalie was born shortly afterward. The family returned to Minneapolis in 1912 so Gustavus could join his brothers in their printing business as well as to be near family. Gustavus became a naturalized American citizen in 1898. He worked as a printer until he died of lung cancer in 1925, which was believed to have been caused by his long history of smoking. Ida was a homemaker all of her life and kept the books for her husband's business. She and Rosalie lived together following her husband's death. She suffered from high blood pressure most of her life and died of cardiac complications in 1957.

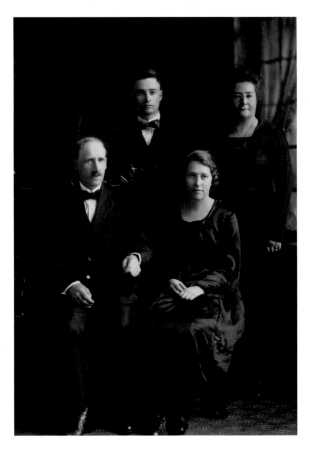

FAMILY BACKGROUND

Rosalie and her brother grew up in the Swedish community of south Minneapolis, and both became fluent in reading and speaking Swedish. Involvement in the Lutheran church was an integral part of family life. Rosalie enjoyed hiking and swimming and continued to pursue these sports throughout her life.

Rosalie attended grade school and high school in Minneapolis and enrolled for one year in the liberal arts program at the University of Minnesota. She soon realized that she wanted to be a nurse and transferred into the newly designated baccalaureate degree program in nursing. She lived at home during college, worked every Saturday to cover college expenses, and described herself as an average student. Her leadership skills began to take shape early, as was evidenced by her involvement in student government in nursing school, first as treasurer and then vice president. She received her nursing degree in June 1924 and a bachelor's degree in Public Health Nursing in March 1925. After working a few years, Rosalie returned to the university in 1932 for a year of course work in premedicine, followed by a year of medical school. At that point, Rosalie realized that she truly wanted to stay in nursing rather than pursue a career in medicine. She left school and returned to a career in public health nursing.

Rosalie's brother, Ralph, chose quite a different career path. He first became a lawyer and a few years later entered divinity school. Upon graduation, he was ordained as a Lutheran pastor. He met and married Ann Marie Peterson (of Danish descent) while serving his first pastorate in South Dakota. They had three sons and one daughter. Ralph died in 1973 of Parkinson's disease. His wife died nine years later of the same disease.

Because she never married, Rosalie spent holidays with Ralph's family, and she always remembered them on special occasions. Her niece, Miriam, said her aunt would send their family postcards from wherever she was working. She also fondly recalls that, when her aunt was working with the American Indians in Arizona, she sent Miriam an Indian doll with a papoose on her back, and while she was in Alaska, Rosalie sent her an Eskimo doll. Miriam credits Rosalie for her interest in nursing as a career.

CAREER PATH
MINNESOTA STATE BOARD OF HEALTH

Rosalie's first job following graduation was with the Minnesota State Board of Health. After the first year, she transferred to a similar position in Minneapolis, which she held for the next four years. New job responsibilities included the supervision of student nurses who were doing their clinical experience as part of the nursing program at the University of Minnesota. Medical school enticed Rosalie away from her nursing career for a brief period of time. In 1934, she returned to public health nursing as the state supervisory nurse in the Division of Child Hygiene at the Minnesota State Health Department. She traveled throughout Minnesota for the next two years fulfilling a variety of duties: inspecting and consulting in Christmas Seal schools for children with handi-

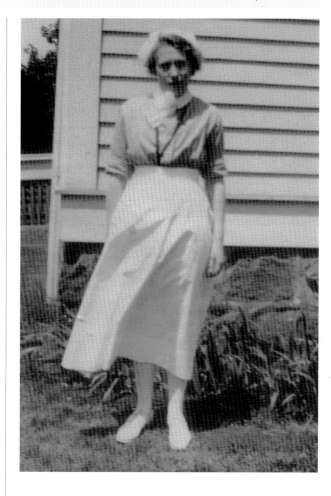

ABOVE
Rosalie Peterson
Student nurse
University of Minnesota
School of Nursing

ROSALIE IRENE PETERSON

BELOW
Rosalie Peterson
Reserve Corps of the U.S.
Public Health Service

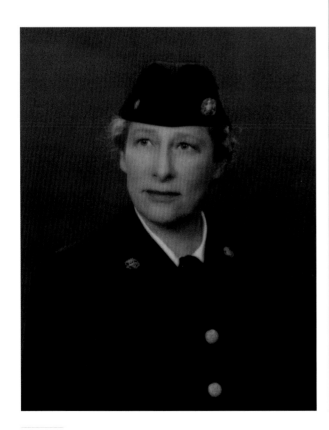

caps, teaching classes to public health nurses, supervising the relief nurses services, and acting as liaison with the State Employment Relations Department.

U.S. PUBLIC HEALTH DEPARTMENT/U.S. INDIAN SERVICE

In 1935, Rosalie moved to Washington DC, where she accepted a position in the U.S. Public Health Service as an assistant public health nursing consultant in scientific research. Two years later, she transferred to the U.S. Indian Service where she planned and directed their public health services. As Rosalie traveled to Indian reservations throughout the country, she brought with her a fervor for delivering a message of cancer prevention and early detection. She was convinced that the public health nurse was key to educating people about changing their smoking, drinking, and eating habits and worked tirelessly at teaching public health nurses ways to bring this message to their clients on the reservations. Her direct approach about such things as smoking and drinking was truly a bold step in those years. Rosalie was not shy about her agenda.

In 1941, Rosalie went back to the U.S. Public Health Service as a nursing consultant. Her new office in New York required that she and her mother move their home from Washington, DC, to Long Island. In her new position, Rosalie consulted with public health nursing directors in 10 states located in the Northeast. This position gave her numerous opportunities to promote her cancer control message. After a short time in this position, her role expanded to include directing public health nursing activities throughout the U.S. Public Health Service. Once again, Rosalie was traveling throughout the United States. Margaret Sheehen, the Director of Nurses at the University of Minnesota Hospital, vividly recalls the visits that Rosalie would make to the hospital and her recommendations for including topics on cancer control in the curriculum for staff development. Rosalie based these recommendations on her belief that teaching nurses at the staff level in the hospital setting as well as in the community was key to early diagnoses. Margaret described Rosalie as being very tactful and approachable whenever she made a site visit and never demanding. To quote Margaret, "Everyone liked her and appreciated her ideas."

In 1945, Rosalie applied for and received a commission in the Reserve Corps of the U.S. Public Health Service. She remained in a civil service capacity within the Public Health Service throughout the war but would have been called to active duty should the situation have warranted it. She received the American Theater Ribbon and a World War II Ribbon in recognition of her active duty in a nonmilitary role in the Public Health Service. Her tour of duty officially was terminated in July 1952.

Simultaneous with serving in the Public Health Reserve Corps, Rosalie carried out her duties as assistant chief at the Office of Public Health Nursing of the U.S. Public Health Service. In the

1948 article "Public Health Nursing in the Cancer Control Program of the U.S. Public Health Service," Rosalie outlined an ambitious program using recently allocated federal dollars for grants-in-aid to states for special projects in cancer control. The first emphasis of these nursing grants was to extend knowledge in cancer within the nursing profession. Secondly, teaching materials were to be developed for students in the basic public health nursing program and for basic nursing schools. To help states with organizing, operating, and directing these cancer programs, Rosalie guided the Public Health Service to give a special orientation in cancer to a small group of public health consultants who, in turn, would be assigned to states (by request) for up to one year. The ultimate goal of this federally funded cancer-control project was better case findings and reduced delays in treatment.

NATIONAL INSTITUTES OF HEALTH/NATIONAL CANCER INSTITUTE

In May 1947, Rosalie accepted the position of chief of the nursing section in the Cancer Control Subdivision at the National Institutes of Health (NIH) in Bethesda, MD, joining the staff for which she already had served as chief public health nursing consultant. She was responsible for planning, organizing, and developing a cancer program that would better prepare nurses through improved teaching of cancer in both basic and advanced professional schools of nursing. To prepare herself for this role, she attended on-the-job training at Roswell Park Memorial Hospital in Buffalo, NY, and at Memorial Hospital in New York City. She increased her knowledge base in cancer care as well as established a professional network with nursing colleagues employed in the cancer hospital setting. These same nurses were among those who would assist Rosalie in future cancer control projects at the National Cancer Institute (NCI).

Rosalie, recognizing her need for further education, took a leave of absence from her position in 1949 and enrolled in the graduate program at Catholic University in Washington, DC, where, in 1950, she earned a master's of science degree in Nursing Education. Her dissertation, "An Analysis of the Cancer Case Load of the Nonofficial Nursing Agency Rendering Bedside Nursing Service in the Home in a Large Metropolitan City," provided data to public health administrators for appraising the cost and scope of a cancer nursing service. Analysis was performed on (a) the cancer case load in relation to the total load, (b) the relationship between the patient with cancer and the patient who is chronically ill, (c) patients who most often are referred for nursing care according to age, sex, and sites of illness, (d) sources of referrals, (e) average length of time patients needed nursing service, (f) frequency of visits, (g) average time of visits, and (h) type of nursing service needed. Study implications included the need for in-service education in cancer care, a need for which Rosalie had long been an advocate.

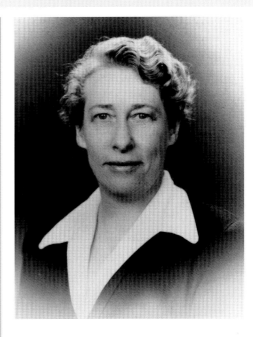

ABOVE
Rosalie Peterson

ROSALIE IRENE PETERSON

BELOW
Rosalie Peterson (first row center left) and Katherine Nelson (first row center right)
National Cancer Institute
Washington, DC, 1949

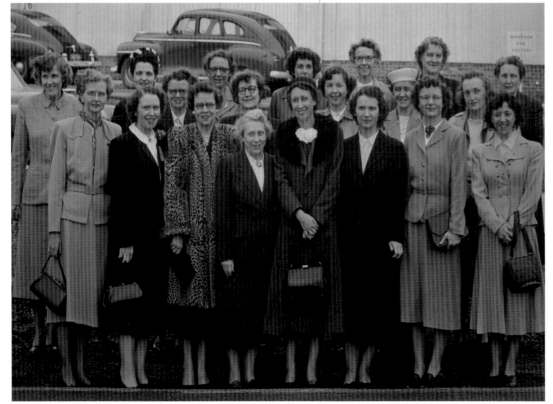

Rosalie returned to NIH and was appointed as chief of the nursing section of the Cancer Control Branch of NCI, which later in the 1950s became the Field Investigation and Demonstration Branch. Rosalie continued to hold this post until her retirement in 1964. Her initiatives led to the development of educational and administrative tools for instructors in universities, schools of nursing, and public health agencies. One of Rosalie's first undertakings, along with Genevieve Soller, assistant chief of the nursing section, was the preparation of the manual *Cancer Nursing in the Basic Professional Nursing Curriculum*. A production team consisting of representatives of nursing education and nursing service was convened in response to numerous requests from instructors for assistance in planning experiences dealing with cancer nursing and activities for students. This group of experts outlined concepts about cancer, cancer nursing, cancer control, and resources for obtaining information. They applied a problem-solving approach in presenting the core content to enhance students' understanding of the complete care of the patient with cancer, including the public health aspects of prevention, early detection, diagnosis, treatment, home care, and rehabilitation. The manual addressed the needs of patients with cancer and their families across the entire cancer continuum.

Rosalie also became the project director for five federally funded projects to integrate cancer nursing into the basic professional nursing curriculum. These grants provided the first monies that were directed at schools of nursing. Skidmore College received one of the grants, which led to Rosalie meeting and working with faculty member Doris Diller, who implemented the Skidmore grant. One of the outcomes of the grant was Diller's development of the Cancer Knowledge Test. In 1957, NCI published another book, *Tools for Evaluation of Cancer Nursing for Nursing Instruction*, under the direction of Rosalie.

In her years at NCI, Rosalie's leadership skills forged partnerships with the American Cancer Society, the federal government, and a number of universities. Katherine Nelson, faculty member at Columbia University in New York City, recalled bringing her entire class of advanced clinical students to Washington for a visit to NCI and the impact this exposure to cancer made on them.

Rosalie responded to requests to provide consultations in France, England, Scotland, Scandinavian countries, Netherlands, and Belgium. In particular, she was asked to give assistance to programs in breast cancer rehabilitation. At one point, upon returning home from France, she began asking questions about why American women always had mastectomies for breast cancer, when in France, a lumpectomy was the treatment of choice.

Several universities and organizations recognized Rosalie with awards for her outstanding service and leadership. Among them were Skidmore College, the American Public Health Association, and the School of Nursing at the University of Minnesota.

Skidmore College

Rosalie I. Peterson, distinguished leader in the field of cancer nursing, you have made outstanding contributions as a public health nurse and educator. In these capacities, you have achieved a high reputation for your devoted and unwavering endeavor to maintain the health of people and to improve the care of patients with cancer.

In recognition of the prominent place you hold in the esteem of your colleagues, Skidmore College, and its Department of Nursing is pleased to add their tribute in the form of this citation.

**SKIDMORE COLLEGE DEPARTMENT OF NURSING
NEW YORK, NEW YORK
January 18, 1957**

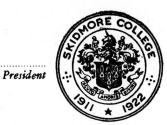

....
President   *Chairman of Department of Nursing*

Dear Irene:

[handwritten letter]

Sincerely, Rosalie.

Upon retirement from her position at NCI, Rosalie received the following letter from Dr. Kenneth Endicott, director of NCI. His words clearly express the impact that Rosalie's contributions made in cancer nursing.

I convey to you my sincere thanks for your completely unselfish and altruistic service to the NCI during your assignment with us. In particular, I should like to commend you for your outstanding contributions in the field of cancer nursing and education. . . . Your efforts have undoubtedly provided a design and purposefulness to the professional life of nurses throughout the country interested in the cancer problem.

RETIREMENT

Following retirement, Rosalie knew she wanted to move out of the Washington, DC, area. She considered the Midwest, where her brother and his children were all living, but preferred the warmth of the Southwest. She bought a home in Sun City, AZ, close to her good friend and nurse colleague, Margaret Knapp.

Rosalie soon became involved in community activities. She knew about the Meals on Wheels program from her Public Health Service days and set about initiating the program in Sun City. This service, designed to improve the nutritional needs of senior citizens, is still a very vital program there today. She also became an active member in a local Lutheran Church and was a willing volunteer when it came to any of their community outreach programs.

In the 1970s, a detached retina left Rosalie blind in one eye. In 1984, she fell in her home, dislocating both shoulders and fracturing the left one. After this, she decided to move to the Good Shepherd Retirement Center. She continued to be mentally sharp and worried about everyone else but herself. In June 1985, she developed shingles, which led to a nonhealing vascular lesion of her leg that required going into isolation in the hospital. Surgical intervention did not alter her condition, which progressed to septicemia and coma. Her niece, Miriam, who also lived in Sun City, was with her during those last days. She recalled her last visit with Rosalie:

"My aunt pulled down my isolation mask, looked at me, smiled and said, 'Thank you, honey.'"

Shortly afterward, Rosalie slipped into a coma. The family decided to move her back to the nursing home where, the following week, she died peacefully on July 8 at the age of 85.

SUMMARY

When Rosalie retired in 1964, she had spent more than 40 years advocating for cancer education and the nurse's role in disseminating the message of cancer control. She had the reputation of being small (5' 2") but mighty. She was not afraid to state her beliefs when she felt strongly about something and was not intimidated by rank or protocol. If something important about nursing should be heard, she made certain that it was. Perhaps Rosalie's boldness made nurses begin to recognize the role they could play in cancer control activities. University schools of nursing began receiving grants to integrate cancer education into their academic curriculum. Rosalie was truly a pioneer in moving cancer nursing forward at a time when nurses were taught very little about cancer, especially in the area of cancer prevention and early detection. Katherine Nelson had this to say about her colleague.

"Rosalie was attentive to the social implications of the whole spectrum of cancer. She was a charming person whose heart was in cancer care, and she was in the heart of the government agencies for cancer, a pivotal position for making change in nursing."

REFERENCES

Peterson, R. (1948). Public health nursing in the cancer control program of the U.S. Public Health Service. *Public Health Nurse, 40,* 74–77.

Peterson, R. (1950). *An analysis of the cancer case load of the Nonofficial Nursing Agency rendering bedside nursing service in the home in a large metropolitan city.* Unpublished master's thesis, Catholic University School of Nursing, Washington, DC.

Peterson, R. (1956). Federal grants for education in cancer nursing, *Nursing Outlook, 4*(2), 103–105.

Interviews by Judith Johnson: niece, Miriam Grunstrup; nephew, James Peterson; and nursing colleagues Margaret Sheehen, Katherine Nelson, Renilda Hilkemeyer, and Doris Diller, March 1999.

Personnel records provided by Public Health Service Historian: John Parascandola, Rockville, MD, and NIH Historian: Victoria Harden, Bethesda, MD.

Documents from Nursing Department Records, Department of Special Collections, Lucy Scribner Library, Skidmore College, Saratoga Springs, NY.

SELECTED WRITINGS

CANCER NURSING IN THE BASIC PROFESSIONAL NURSING CURRICULUM (1951)

The Problem

Most informed people recognize cancer as a major public health problem today and appreciate the need for more effective education and control. It is the second chief cause of death in the Nation. The Cancer Control Branch of the National Cancer Institute states that the increase in the cancer morbidity rate between 1937 and 1947 was 34 percent. Even when the effects of the aging population are taken into account there remains a residual increase of 27 percent in the morbidity rate.

It is estimated that the number of new cases of cancer will be as follows: 524,000 in 1950, 570,000 in 1955, and 675,000 in 1965.

Since cancer is a silent disease and does not manifest itself by an explosive onset, there will be a large number of persons in the population who will have the disease without knowledge of its existence.

Cancer appears in all age groups, but 84 percent of the cases occur in individuals over 45 years of age. It is a disease that is costly to diagnose and to treat. Many communities are without diagnostic or treatment facilities or public health nursing service. These factors contribute to the high cancer morbidity and mortality rates.

Every general hospital gives care to cancer patients and it is likely that the number of patients will increase as facilities for early discovery are made available. In a typical 250-bed hospital, which for purposes of discussion is assumed to be constantly filled, one can expect that 13 beds will be occupied exclusively by cancer patients. Out of a total of 9,000 admissions during a year, 225 will be for cancer. About half of the cases will be admitted in an advanced-stage of the disease. The average length of stay will be 21 days for the cancer patient as compared with an average of 7 days for other hospital patients. The treatment will be for curative and palliative purposes.

The patient with cancer requires continuous medical supervision after his hospital discharge. Many patients will be discovered early and achieve cures. Others will pass into the terminal stage. No national studies have been made to ascertain where terminal care is given; however, it is estimated that 50 percent will receive this care outside the hospital. Many of these will remain in their own homes, while others will be cared for in nursing homes, county homes, and other public institutions. The problem of meeting the needs of these patients is apparent.

Most cancer patients require skilled nursing care at some time during their illness. Today one-third of the patients with cancer are being cured. It is believed that if present diagnostic and curative services were available to everyone and were used, another one-third of the people who develop cancer could be saved, and useful, productive lives could be prolonged for many. There is a marked lag between knowledge and action.

Cancer in the Curriculum

Nursing educators recognize that if the curriculum is to fulfill its purpose, it must be based on the needs of society as well as the needs of the student. For qualitative nursing education, student experiences will be broad and include the hospital, home, school, occupational environment, and community. The study of any disease will embrace health promotion, diagnosis, and treatment including nursing care, rehabilitation, and the relationships of this disease to others.

The Cancer Content Production Committee acknowledges that cancer is but one disease with which the nurse must be competent to deal, and that there are many ways of teaching disease entities. However, it is the consensus that cancer nursing should not be taught as a special course but integrated with such courses as nursing arts, pediatrics, gynecology, obstetrics, medical-surgical nursing, and public health. The consideration of cancer in relation to other illnesses enlarges the opportunities for the student to learn likeness and difference in symptoms, diagnostic procedures, treatment, and nursing care. Emphasis on the similarity of problems offers the opportunity to guide the student in developing a better appreciation of the social, emotional, and economic implications of all illness.

To accomplish integration, instructors will need to work together to set up objectives, outline total content, and plan related activities. Frequent meetings will be needed to report progress and to check the "total plan" outline of instruction to prevent duplications and omissions.

Planning the sequence of learning experiences is the prerogative of the teacher. Helpful criteria for selecting these experiences are:

1. Nature of the problem. 2. Increasing difficulty of the subject matter. 3. Amount of growth the experience will provide. 4. Readiness of the learner for the experience. Too much emphasis cannot be placed on this latter point as far as cancer is concerned. Because of previous life experiences, many students may have developed undesirable attitudes toward cancer before coming to the school of nursing. Selection of experiences emphasizing patients with more favorable prognosis is recommended as a means of assisting in the improvement of attitudes.

Cancer nursing experiences for student nurses should take place not only in the hospital but in the tumor clinics and other clinics, homes, health departments, and welfare agencies. The school of nursing is responsible for the quality and amount of education and supervision of the students' experience through selection of such agencies, joint planning, payment of tuition fees, and periodic revaluation of the experience. The agency providing the experience must understand the objectives of the educational program of the school of nursing and the role the agency is to play, and must provide competent supervision.

Note. From *Cancer Nursing in the Basic Professional Nursing Curriculum* (Public Health Service Publication No. 147) by National Cancer Institute of the National Institutes of Health, 1951, Washington, DC: U.S. Government Printing Office.

ROSALIE IRENE PETERSON

PUBLIC HEALTH NURSING IN THE CANCER CONTROL PROGRAM OF THE U.S. PUBLIC HEALTH SERVICE (1948)

Those of us who are older public health nurses, whenever we think of the cancer patient, will probably call to mind the extremely ill patients such as we cared for as student nurses. Their suffering was probably the most excruciating endured by any patient. We may also think of the odors that made it so repulsive to be with the patient. If that is your mental picture of cancer patients, I hope that you will have an opportunity to visit a hospital today where such patients are looked after. One seldom sees the patient who is suffering the excruciating pain that was common in the earlier days. In fact very little morphine is given to patients. Palliative surgery is now done, regardless of the age of patients. Persons who are in the 80's have such radical surgery as complete gastrectomy, whole lungs are removed, rectums are removed, radical surgery on the face is done and new faces are fashioned. In most hospitals where such radical surgery is done, the patients are given highly concentrated diets with huge amounts of vitamins. Plasma is given prior to surgery, and whole blood and plasma are given following surgery. At an early period, patients are taught to take care of themselves. Colostomy patients are taught to take an enema sometimes daily and sometimes every other day, and very often the body regulates itself to having a normal bowel movement once daily. Colostomy dressings in some institutions consist only of paper tissues worn under a two-way stretch garment. When stomachs are removed, the intestines soon modify the function and assume those of the stomach also, and . . . the patients get along on three meals a day. Patients who have had tracheotomies are taught to rinse the inner tube as frequently as needed and in some institutions are taught to remove the outer tube also. Patients who have had radical facial surgery have new noses, new ears, and new faces built either by plastic surgery or a prosthesis in our hospitals today.

However even more important are some of the methods of early diagnosis that are being developed. Some of you have already heard of, and all of you will soon know of the Papanicolaou test, or, as the test will soon be called, CTC (cytologic test for cancer). The test is a simple smear which may be obtained from excretions from the cervix and body of the uterus or may be made from fluids or aspirated materials from other parts of the body, spread on a microscopic slide and properly fixed and sent to a laboratory for a special staining, the Papanicolaou stain. This stain shows cells which have undergone nuclear change. Although it takes trained pathologists or technicians to make the stain and to read the slides, the family physician is able to make the smear in his office when the patient reports for examination, and he then mails the slide to a laboratory for a report. Think what this will mean in early detection of cancer, especially of the genital tract.

Note. From "Public Health Nursing in the Cancer Control Program of the U.S. Public Health Service," by R. Peterson, 1948, *Public Health Nursing, 40,* pp. 76–77. Copyright 1948 by Blackwell Science, Inc. Excerpted with permission.

TRIBUTES

Rosalie Peterson was an administrator, educator, author, and cancer nursing expert. She was concerned about nurses' lack of knowledge about cancer, cancer nursing, home care and rehabilitation, and the belief that cancer always was fatal. She started a multifaceted program to change the outlook of nurses and improve the care of patients with cancer and became actively involved in causes and courses for cancer nursing. She taught cancer care to public health nurses and, in 1948, awarded grants to the University of Minnesota and Columbia University to enrich their graduate curriculum. In 1950, Rosalie and two other members of her staff conducted a three-week Institute in Cancer Nursing for 30 instructors across the country at the University of Minnesota. I was one of those instructors.

Rosalie was ahead of her time. She tried to get cancer nursing recognized as a specialty in graduate nursing programs. However, this period, 1948–1950, was the era of generalization, not specialization, so the project was not successful nationwide. Rosalie did not let the lack of graduate education in cancer nursing deter her in her major goal of increasing knowledge in cancer nursing education and improving the care of patients with cancer. She became legendary when she funded five pilot programs for cancer education to integrate cancer nursing at the baccalaureate level. As a result of these programs, Doris Diller developed a cancer knowledge test at Skidmore College, a curriculum for cancer in the basic curriculum, a professional nursing curriculum, and tools to evaluate cancer nursing for nursing instructors. These cancer nursing programs in the baccalaureate-degree schools of nursing had an impact on cancer nursing and the care of patients with cancer.

Starting in the 1950s, Rosalie and her staff contributed a great deal to the nursing literature about public health and nursing education. In cooperation with the New York State Health Department, she published a manual, *Cancer Nursing and Cancer*, in 1963. This booklet included epidemiologic information as well as nursing care aspects. In 1973, a manual for public health nurses followed the booklet. Rosalie also was a member of the first Nursing Advisory Committee of the American Cancer Society chaired by Katherine Nelson.

I was honored to have Rosalie as a colleague, mentor, and friend. One day in 1950, when I was conducting a program in cancer nursing for public health nurses at the Ellis Fischel State Cancer Hospital, I received a call from the Regional Public Health Nurse Officer who said that the Director of Programs from the National Cancer Institute, Rosalie Peterson, wanted to see what I was doing. I liked Rosalie during our initial contact. She stood at about 5' 2" and had short, white hair and steel-blue, penetrating eyes. In 1952, she appointed me as a special consultant to the section of the Field Investigations and Demonstration Branch. I was involved in meetings, conferences, and educational programs. She was quick to introduce me as a clinically competent expert in cancer nursing. She

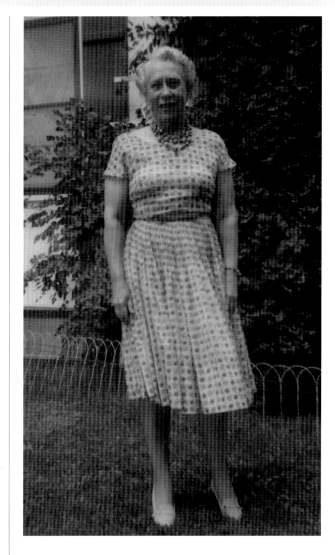

ABOVE
Rosalie Peterson

used her position, talents, and zeal for cancer nursing. She was influential as a significant contributor to upgrading cancer nursing practice through educational programs and literature.

Rosalie was the inspiration for my going to M.D. Anderson Hospital as the Director of Nursing. She referred me to R. Lee Clark, MD, Director and Surgeon in Chief of the University of Texas M. D. Anderson Hospital and Tumor Institute, who had sought Rosalie to help him find a Director of Nursing for his new hospital. After I was at M.D. Anderson for a while, Rosalie visited the University of Texas in Galveston to see about setting up a graduate program in cancer nursing using M.D. Anderson as a clinical area. Unfortunately, there was no interest.

Rosalie visited me unofficially. She met my mother, who had a chronic heart problem. When Rosalie learned that my mother wanted to see Washington, DC, she took over that project with the same zest as her work. She planned the touring, breaks, and rest periods. We had a delightful time. I have very fond memories. I admire the contributions Rosalie made to cancer nursing and feel privileged to have collaborated with her.

Renilda Hilkemeyer, RN, BS, DPS

I first met Rosalie in January of 1950. I was invited, as a faculty member from one of 24 educational institutions, to a three-week course in cancer nursing. The course was held at the University of Minnesota, which was Rosalie's alma mater. She made very sure that we were taught all aspects of prevention and early detection and how to integrate this into our curriculum at our schools. The expectation was to teach every student breast self-exam. This may seem commonplace now, but back then, in 1950, this idea was revolutionary.

Rosalie made frequent visits to Skidmore in New York City. This was partly because she was overseeing our grant. We all liked her; she was kind, interested in others, and asked good questions. Yet, at the same time, she expected people to get things done!

Rosalie was my houseguest on several occasions. When I think back to that time, I can't recall ever talking with her about anything except nursing. Nursing was her passion! Within nursing, her goal was to have cancer nursing clearly identified and understood within nursing education. To this end, she secured grants for us, held faculty summer institutes, and strove to provide continuing education for all nurses. She always wanted prevention and early detection to be part of every educational effort.

One interesting note that I can add is that, for a time, Rosalie lived across the hall from J. Edgar Hoover. We used to wonder who she met coming and going and figured she had some good stories to tell!

We were very fortunate to have Rosalie at the National Institutes of Health (NIH). When she arrived there, nursing was on the bottom rung of the ladder. Rosalie knew how to network in Washington and where to garner support for her ideas. She quickly gained respect among her medical colleagues at NIH. She would not hesitate to call us when she needed advice or counsel. Rosalie had a job to do, and she spent the rest of her professional career doing just that. When she retired from NIH, nursing had moved up the ladder to a much more visible position. We were receiving grants, were on review boards, were being ask to make site visits, and, in general, nurses were being respected for their contributions in cancer. We have Rosalie to thank for setting us on an upward path.

Doris Diller, RN, MA

Professional papers and effects of Rosalie Peterson are located in the archives at the National Office of the Oncology Nursing Society in Pittsburgh, PA.

KATHERINE R. NELSON, RN, BS, MA, EdD
Leader in Cancer Nursing Education

"Looking back, I can see clearly now that (in so many things that I have accomplished) I was the facilitator or expediter. Others thought up the idea, and I was called on to do the work . . . to make it work."

— Katherine R. Nelson

KATHERINE R. NELSON

SIGNIFICANT CAREER CONTRIBUTIONS

- Developed questions for the first national test pool for the state board examinations in nursing

- One of the first nurses to hold a joint appointment as a college faculty member and director of hospital nursing education

- Developed the first university-based advanced clinical course in cancer nursing for graduate nurses

- First Chair of the American Cancer Society (ACS) National Nursing Advisory Committee

- First nurse awarded the ACS National Distinguished Service Award

- Initiated the first course in cancer nursing at the university level, offering master's and doctoral degrees in clinical specialization

---

BIOGRAPHICAL INFORMATION

BIRTH

Katherine Rose Nelson was born on October 11, 1907, in Waterbury, CT.

PARENTS

Katherine was one of five daughters born to Charles and Margaret (Butler) Nelson, three of whom became nurses. Her only brother died at the age of two. Her father, who was born in Sweden, was a foreman at a brass manufacturing company in Waterbury. Katherine attributes the origin of her own administrative and management skills to the influence and example set by her father, a manager highly respected by those who worked for him as well as by his peers. Katherine's mother, Margaret, was the daughter of Irish-English immigrant parents. She was a homemaker, busy throughout the day with the multiple tasks of a large family. Katherine recalled that her mother always was baking, cooking, cleaning, laundering, and sewing clothes for the family. Katherine also remembered eating her first piece of "bought" bread at the age of 10 and purchasing her first "store-bought" dress after she finished high school.

FAMILY

Katherine's childhood was one of great freedom and flexibility. She had freedom from the pervasive violence that is in today's youth culture, and "sex, drugs, and violence" were all but unknown in the early 1900s. She also believed that the curiosity, flexibility, and creativity one is born with have to be nurtured during childhood, as it was for the Nelson children. Preoccupation with electronic games and television was not an issue. Instead, children were sent out to play, and, in doing so, became very creative and inventive, all the while learning to interact with others. Katherine did not recognize until many years later that her childhood gave her that freedom, creativity, and flexibility that characterized her professional life. She feels fortunate "to have been born at a very good time."

Her siblings are Florence Boulanger, who was a nurse's aide with the Red Cross at Waterbury Hospital in Connecticut during World War II and is deceased; Margaret Boandl, RN, who worked at St. Luke's Hospital in Bethlehem, PA, and currently resides in New Mexico; Ruth Nelson, RN, who was a lieutenant in the U.S. Army Nurses Corp during World War II and worked at Columbia Presbyterian and Women's Hospital in New York, who currently resides in Waterbury; and Evelyn Nelson, who served in the Women's Army Corps in Africa and Italy and was decorated with the Bronze Star for her work in military communications, who is deceased.

CAREER PATH

Katherine's parents had a strong influence on her career. She wanted to be a teacher, but her parents discouraged her from attending the classical high school that would have prepared her to pursue a teaching career. Instead, she took commercial courses with the intent of going to work after graduation. At her mother's suggestion, Katherine enrolled at Pratt Institute in Brooklyn, NY, to study dietetics, graduating two years later with a certificate. This was an emerging field at the time, and Katherine readily obtained a position at St. Francis Hospital in Hartford, CT, as the only dietitian in the 500-bed hospital. She received full room and board plus $25 per week. Although she never married, her social life was quite full. During the Roaring Twenties, Katherine, the "flapper," entered and won an endurance dance contest.

After five years of watching trays leave the kitchen full and return empty, Katherine was "bored pink" with the monotony of the job. In her role as a dietitian, Katherine had frequent opportunities to observe the nurses in their varied and interesting roles throughout the hospital setting. She decided to change directions and study nursing, which looked like a much more stimulating and exciting field than dietetics. In l933, she enrolled in the School of Nursing at The Johns Hopkins Hospital, choosing that program because of the research being conducted on vitamins and nutrition. Entering nurse's training at that time took great courage. Unemployment was rampant during the Depression, and nurses were offering to work in hospitals without pay in exchange for three meals a day.

JOHNS HOPKINS HOSPITAL

During her three years in nursing school, Katherine "kept waiting to be told what nursing was, and the only thing they told me was what nurses did (i.e., the procedures)." Her first job upon graduation was that of head nurse on the Metabolism Research Ward, a position she was offered because of her combined nursing and dietetics background. Katherine coauthored an article on desoxy-corticosterones with two research scientists from Hopkins, which was published in *Lancet* in 1938.

While still the head nurse, Katherine was asked to explore the teaching methods and content of the dietetics curriculum for nurses and dietetics students. She spent two weeks visiting other major teaching hospitals in the Northeast, returning to Hopkins with a new approach to curriculum design. Katherine moved the dietetics students out of the kitchen and onto the wards to meet and study patients with nutritional problems. She also designed an appetite chart to be used by student nurses as a teaching tool with their patients, freeing the students from their former roles in food preparation.

Katherine spent the next three years as a supervisor and clinical instructor at Johns Hopkins. As America was gearing up for World War II, Katherine considered joining the Army Nurse Corps along with a friend, Eleanore Niernsee. Her director advised her against it because her value was

Sad as it may seem, I believe nursing has no goals for cancer at all! Yes, nurses wish to help the patient, after the surgeon has performed his radical treatment. And yes, nurses want to help the patient after he's in the late stage of cancer and needs endless convalescent or custodial care. But, that doesn't answer the question! What does nursing want to do about cancer? Well, and as it may seem I would say harshly nothing. *In fact, we want to do something worse; we want to run away and hope that cancer will disappear before we come back.*

NELSON, 1973, P. 141

KATHERINE R. NELSON

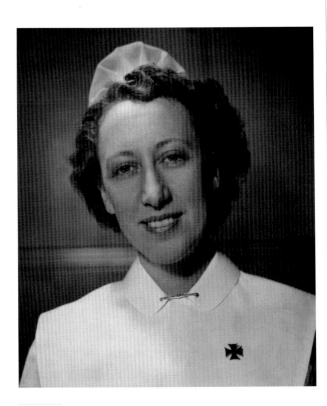

much greater as an instructor who could turn out 20–30 more nurses every year to serve in the military. In 1941, Katherine enrolled in the Teachers College at Columbia University. Her long-held desire to be a teacher was stronger than ever. "I knew that my vocation was teaching. It was not nursing; it was not dietetics; it was teaching." She graduated with a bachelor's of science degree in 1942, with a major in clinical teaching and supervision.

HARTFORD HOSPITAL

Following graduation from Columbia, Katherine went to work at Hartford Hospital in Connecticut as a medical supervisor. She also prepared the supplies and nursing volunteers for immediate response in the event of an enemy attack on the vulnerable East Coast. The military demand for nurses was great, but long delays occurred between graduation and eligibility for practice because each state had to write, administer, and grade its own licensure examination. Dr. R. Louise McManus from the Teachers College asked Katherine to return to New York in 1943 to participate in a project of the National League for Nursing Education, which was intended to help break the bottleneck resulting from the cumbersome state licensing process. Along with Dr. McManus, Katherine and two colleagues, Phyllis Sammul and Ida Sommer, spent the summer of 1943 writing questions for the first national test pool for state board examinations.

TEACHERS COLLEGE IN COLUMBIA

Katherine accepted a teaching position at the Teachers College at Columbia University as an instructor in nursing education. She earned a master's degree in Administration of Schools of Nursing from the Teachers College in 1945. She briefly entertained the possibility of accepting a nursing faculty position at Wayne State University in Detroit, MI. However, after visiting the Detroit campus, the New Englander decided that because the position was no different from the one she held at Columbia, she would rather remain in the familiar and traditional campus setting of the Northeast.

During a discussion of faculty and curriculum changes that took place as the war came to an end, Dr. McManus mentioned needing someone for a "cancer program." Katherine readily acknowledged, "That's when I opened my mouth and put my whole future into it!" Katherine's query—"What's the cancer thing?"—opened the door to her distinguished career as an innovative cancer nursing educator and an advocate for the recognition of cancer nursing as a specialty. The Memorial Hospital for Cancer and Allied Diseases in New York City had received a $30,000 grant from the American Cancer Society (ACS) to establish an advanced clinical course in cancer nursing for graduate nurses. Anne Ferris, Director of Nursing at Memorial Hospital, recognized the importance of a university-based course and approached Teachers College to establish a joint program. Dr. McManus thought Katherine had the necessary talents ("freedom, flexibility, and creativity") to create such a program and urged her to accept the challenge. That challenge came from several directions. When Dr. Cornelius Rhoads, Director of Memorial Hospital, interviewed Katherine regarding her suitability for the faculty position, he openly challenged her lack of experience in cancer nursing. Dr. Rhoads indicated that it would make more sense to select a nurse from one of Memorial's units who knew all about cancer to handle the program. Katherine's retort was typically direct as she said, "Of course she knows cancer, but you either have to take a well-prepared cancer nurse and teach her nursing education, or you have to take a person of my qualifications and background in education and teach me cancer nursing. Dr. Rhoads, the decision is yours."

Katherine was appointed as instructor in nursing education at the Teachers College and director of nursing education at Memorial Hospital. She immediately immersed herself in learning all aspects of cancer and cancer nursing. She spent months working and observing throughout the hospital, attending conferences and lectures, and developing the nursing curriculum. The advanced clinical program in cancer nursing (the first in the world) admitted its first students in February 1947, offering a one-year, 16 credit-hour program applicable toward a master's of arts degree. The courses were very comprehensive, covering in-depth studies of cancer as a disease, care of patients with varied cancer di-

BELOW
Katherine Nelson (far right) with the first group of students enrolled in the first advanced program in clinical nursing Memorial Hospital for Cancer and Allied Diseases New York 1947

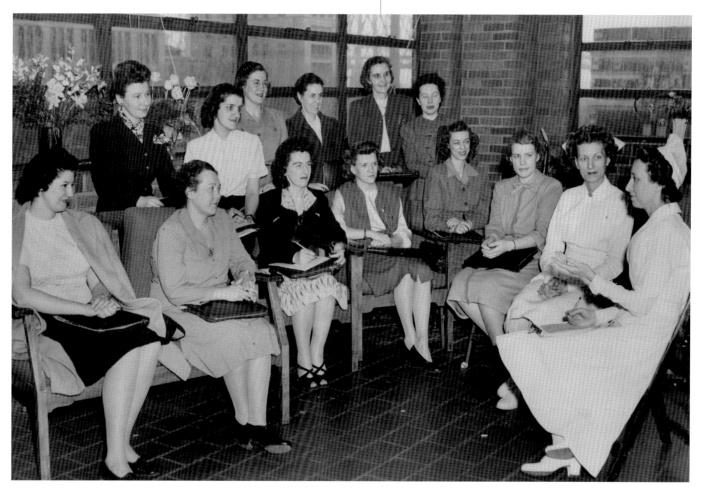

KATHERINE R. NELSON

agnoses, clinic- and community-based experiences, and time spent in terminal-care facilities. Katherine acknowledged the invaluable contributions of Elizabeth Walker, at Memorial Hospital, and Nelliana Best, a public health nurse, for their active roles in ensuring that the students had access to optimal clinical experiences. The program, as originally conceived by Katherine, ran for nearly five years, ending in 1951 when funds were no longer made available. The Teachers College continued to offer a very abbreviated cancer-nursing course; however, the growing trend was to integrate cancer content into general nursing curricula.

When the program ended, Katherine left Teachers College and began what she called "the Nelson improvement program," renewing and strengthening her bedside nursing skills. She worked in the neoplastic wards at Montefiore Hospital in New York City and then with the Public Health Nursing Service in Greenwich, CT. She continued to teach cancer nursing each summer for 14 years (1948–1962) at the University of North Carolina School of Public Health, delineating the public health aspects of cancer in this primarily rural area. She points with pride to the fact that although her classes were segregated by race, she taught the nurses in both groups from identical content material.

Katherine became widely recognized and sought after as an expert on cancer nursing and cancer nursing education. She spoke at many conferences, served on a variety of cancer-related committees, and was appointed as the first chair of ACS's National Nursing Advisory Committee. After serving as assistant director at the Grace-New Haven School of Nursing (1955–1956), Katherine returned to Teachers College to pursue a doctoral degree. In 1960, she was awarded an EdD in Administration of Schools of Nursing. Katherine's academic career then continued at Teachers

BELOW
Katherine Nelson (far right) with first class of African American public health nurses being provided the same course in cancer nursing as white public health nurses received
North Carolina College
Durham
1950

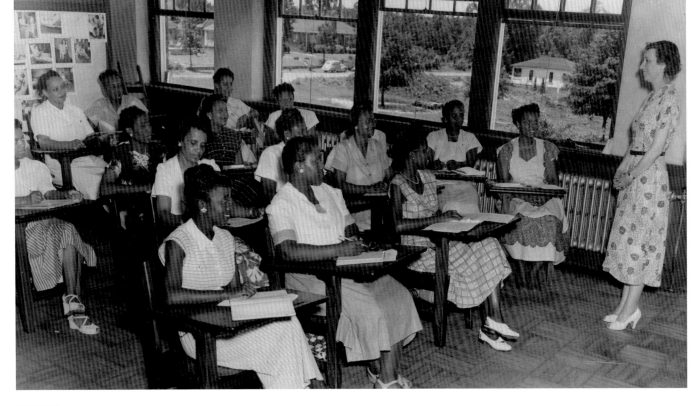

College, first as an assistant professor and then as an associate professor of nursing education. In addition to teaching cancer nursing, she also taught curriculum and research courses in nursing education. Katherine initiated the first course in cancer nursing in the country at the university level at Columbia in 1960. The course offered master's and doctoral degrees in clinical specialization. Katherine became widely known for her tireless effort over the years to gain recognition and acknowledgment of cancer nursing as

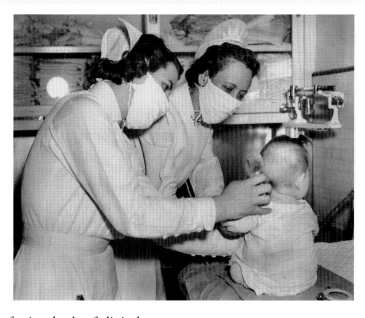

LEFT
Katherine Nelson (right), Director of Nursing Education at Memorial Hospital, with student, Margaret Mead (left), in pediatric ward with baby born with extensive lymphosarcoma of the face
Memorial Hospital
New York

BELOW
Katherine Nelson (front center), National Institute
School of Nursing
Taipei, Taiwan
1967

a specialty, leading to the current professional role of clinical nurse specialist in oncology. Katherine served as advisor to many doctoral candidates and was widely respected for her contributions to their professional development.

During the 1960s, the China Medical Board of New York, Inc. requested Katherine to study the feasibility of establishing a master's degree program in nursing education at the National Taiwan University in Taipei. Her completion of this study led to requests for her to provide consultation services to schools of nursing in the Philippine Islands and in Bangkok, Thailand. In all of these projects, Katherine never failed to emphasize the importance of including cancer in the nursing curriculum. Her international reputation as an educator led to an invitation to conduct an Institute on Nursing Education in Portugal in 1971. The Institute, sponsored by the Catholic Nurses Association of Portugal, took place in Lisbon. Afterward, Katherine was honored with the Francisco Gentil Medal for her work in the improvement of nursing care to patients with cancer.

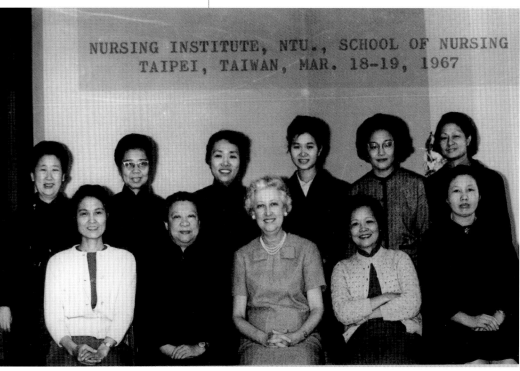

NURSING INSTITUTE, NTU., SCHOOL OF NURSING
TAIPEI, TAIWAN, MAR. 18-19, 1967

KATHERINE R. NELSON

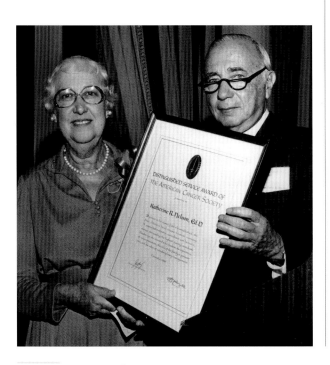

RETIREMENT

Katherine retired from Teachers College in 1972, with the permanent rank of Associate Professor of Nursing Education. She was called upon to serve as an advisor by the fledgling group of cancer nurses who banded together in the early 1970s to form the Oncology Nursing Society. Along with providing advice and wise counsel, Katherine lobbied against the use of the term "oncology" in the organization's name, maintaining steadfastly that we are not nursing "the study of tumors," we are nursing "people with cancer."

In 1974, Katherine was invited to serve as a member of a team sent to South Korea by the Academy of Educational Development in New York City. This team studied the status of education for health professionals, visiting all universities in South Korea. Katherine continued her personal crusade, emphasizing the need for increased awareness of cancer as a major health problem throughout the world and advocating for inclusion of cancer content in nursing education.

After serving as a consultant on curriculum design, Katherine attempted to settle into the social life of retirement but found it quite unsatisfactory. When she was 70 years old, she volunteered for one year as a live-in counselor at Covenant House in New York City, which serves as a refuge for young runaways. Katherine's vivid reflections of her experiences there illustrate the depth of her compassion for people. From the patients with cancer on whom she focused to the nursing students whom she inspired to the elderly relatives for whom she cared, Katherine has been a role model of excellence. She has been the recipient of many honors, including the

- Merit Citation, School of Medicine, National Taiwan University
- Merit Citation, School of Nursing, University of the Philippines
- Achievement Award for Practice, The Nursing Education Alumni Association, Teachers College, Columbia University.

SUMMARY

In 1980, Katherine was selected as the first nurse recipient of ACS's Distinguished Service Award. The following excerpts from the presentation ceremony summarize the breadth and depth of her multiple contributions to cancer nursing education and patient care.

"Dr. Katherine Nelson is a nurse educator whose long and distinguished career has been devoted to cancer. A pioneer in the field, she was the first nurse teaching at the university level to insist that cancer nursing was a specialty that must be learned with both theory and clinical practicum

at the master's level. Her introduction of such a course at Columbia University was a milestone and soon was accepted as a model by schools of nursing offering advanced preparation in oncology. It included emphasis on research, teaching, and consultation at a time when the nursing role was largely restricted to patient care. Many of Dr. Nelson's former students occupy leadership positions in cancer nursing today, for she was a forceful motivator, relentless in her demands for excellence in performance.

". . . She urged nurses to perceive their role in the prevention of cancer, to combine teaching with service, to include families of patients and the public in their areas of concern, to recognize the devastating impact of cancer, to insist on a broader scientific base in their teaching, and to work cooperatively with all disciplines.

"One of the first nurse consultants in cancer, Katherine Nelson's tremendous energy and enthusiasm were communicated to thousands of colleagues throughout the country. She gave tirelessly of her time to support cancer nursing projects and plans. Her dedication became legendary as she worked here and abroad, always urging professionalism in nursing as an author, teacher, and role model."

REFERENCES

Nelson, K.R. (1973). The future of cancer nursing. *Proceedings of the National Conference on Cancer Nursing, USA*, 141–145.

Nelson, K.R. (1987). *The history of cancer in the nursing curriculum, 1860–1951. Proceedings: Cancer nurses make it happen: A tenth anniversary history of the nursing committee.* Wallingford, CT: American Cancer Society, Connecticut Division.

Nelson, Katherine, interview by Laura Hilderley, March 1999.

KATHERINE R. NELSON

SELECTED WRITING

THE HISTORY OF CANCER IN THE NURSING CURRICULUM, 1860–1951
(1987)

(In the first paragraphs of this paper, Dr. Nelson discusses the evolution of nursing education from the apprenticeship method of the 1860s to the founding of hospital schools of nursing in the United States in the 1870s.)

As students spread to the various wards of the hospital, instruction soon evolved to help students function more effectively in the different wards. Medical nursing dealt with conditions encountered on the medical wards, surgical nursing for conditions encountered on the surgical wards and so on. . . . Apparently no one noticed that there was no instructional harmony in these course titles. Medicine and surgery are really physician's therapies, pediatrics is an age-level designation and obstetrics deals with a normal body process. . . . One finds humorous course titles like *operating room nursing*, and *emergency room nursing!* It is as if someone could nurse an operating room or an emergency room! So much for garbling the English language.

Now that we have said there was no underlying philosophy to the curriculum of schools of nursing up to the time of the 1940's, there really was a central idea that held the whole thing together. That idea was the activities nurses carry out in different locations in a hospital. . . . medical nursing really doesn't exist. To become subject matter for teaching, it has to be translated into types of patient conditions encountered most frequently on medical wards. Interestingly enough, the types of patient conditions encountered most frequently on medical wards are cancer (leukemia and Hodgkin's Disease), heart conditions, diabetes mellitus, all sorts of infections, etc. The same is true of surgical nursing. . . one will encounter patients with cancer, heart disease, diabetes, etc.

But the nurse educators of these early days could not see this. So entrenched was the idea of medical nursing, surgical nursing, orthopedic nursing . . . and so forth, that *this was* the curriculum!

. . . In the late 1930's it was obvious that scientific advances were slowly changing health patterns and that some of the old needs for nursing, such as communicable disease control, were slowly giving way to new needs such as caring for persons with heart disease and persons with cancer. . . . the health professions were beginning to recognize that heart disease and cancer were becoming the "killers" of the future. Efforts were gearing up to cope with them. Nursing educators were quite aware of the emergence of these new health problems but were puzzled as to what to do about it. You couldn't teach a course in cancer nursing if there was no cancer ward in the hospital to which to send the student for practice so what were you to do? It was all a great puzzle. Fortunately . . . a new philosophy in curriculum was being talked about. It was the educational practice known as "integration." According to this idea . . . curriculum remained intact. If a new knowledge or idea appeared on the educational scene it was to be integrated into a well established curriculum offering. Here was the solution! You could leave undisturbed the curriculum oriented to hospital locations. It now seemed quite right and proper to integrate a little cancer instruction into all the well established and familiar courses. Leukemia could go into medical nursing, mastectomies, laryngectomies and radical dissections could go into surgical nursing, Wilm's tumor and retinoblastoma could go into pediatric nursing and so on. Unfortunately in many instances this little became very little indeed and some of the major therapies for cancer were dealt with briefly or left out entirely. A little chemotherapy was put into pharmacology but instruction in radiation as a therapy was practically non-existent. Students knew that patients received radiation therapy but had little knowledge of why or what to do about it. If the patient's physician wanted something done, he left an order to that effect and that was the end of it.

Even though the educational philosophy of integration of subject matter was highly regarded in the 1940s, it left a lot to be desired. One is reminded of the old truism, "what is everybody's business is nobody's business." Unfortunately this was all too true. Every teacher was supposed to be teaching cancer, or any of the other major health deviations, but since no concerted effort was made to check on how well this was being done, it was pretty minimal in many instances.

At this time, although nursing education now felt comfortable about the teaching of cancer and other health deviations, other fields of endeavor in nursing were not so happy. This was especially true of public health nursing agencies. The graduate nurses of the day were wonderfully prepared to be employed in hospitals but when they were employed in a public health agency, it was a different story. They were excellent nursing technicians but they had fairly limited knowledge or appreciation of disease control in society or what was happening to the patient and/or family that was affected by that disease. To cope with this woeful state of affairs, nursing education struggled with long discussions of functional method of assignment versus case method of assignment. Everyone seemed anxious in those days to see the patient as a person, but strangely enough such valiant efforts brought little or no change. The ward work had to be done, students were there to do it and many were advised "don't waste your time talking to the patients!" Unfortunately, the old curriculum remained entrenched and nursing students continued to give much service to the hospitals but were eventually short-changed in the many wider aspects of true professional nursing.

. . . In 1942 The Public Health Nurse Curriculum Guide was published to help colleges or universities which offered graduate programs in public health nursing . . . specifically preparing a graduate nurse who was to be a practitioner of nursing, not a supervisor or administrator of a public health nursing agency . . . Sixteen functional areas were recommended, one of which was CANCER! This in its way is an important historical milestone. To this writer's knowledge, this is the first time

KATHERINE R. NELSON

in nursing education history that a specific part of the program was devoted solely to cancer. It is not buried in some other instructional focus such as medical and surgical nursing. Of course one must be reminded that this is not a course in cancer nursing. It is a recommendation for inclusion of specific subject matter within a course in public health nursing. One might ask: "Well, isn't this the same as integrating cancer into other subject matter?" The answer is no. Instead, cancer is faced head on for what it is, a deviation from normal by human and other forms of life on earth which have a basic biological structure of cells. Humans have cancer, fish have cancer, animals, trees, and other plant life have cancer, and even some dinosaur bones have been dug up which show evidence that the creature had cancer. Looking at subject matter this way is a far cry from the old curriculum way of only providing knowledge that make one's work more efficient.

(Dr. Nelson continues the chronicle of nursing education and curriculum design in the United States from 1940 to the latter half of the 1980s, with emphasis on the changing place of cancer nursing education in both graduate and undergraduate programs.)

We are now in the late 1980's and the 20th century is rapidly waning. To what extent has the curriculum or the practice of nursing progressed since Florence Nightingale's first curriculum for nursing education in 1860? One wonders.

Sadly, this writer feels that nursing education made a serious mistake in the early 1950's when it abandoned its efforts in advanced clinical nursing inquiry, for inquiry into our functions. This opened up a thirty year period of endless academic inquiry on concepts, principles, functions and nursing theory. All of these academic discourses become useless if they do not deal rigorously with two questions: 1) What has happened to the patient in his deviation from health, and 2) How can nursing help him return to health, or to the best use of his remaining capabilities, if total health is not reasonable in his case? This writer feels that it is high time that nursing truly dealt with patients and their needs and not with high flown academic phrases on one hand and expertise on getting the institution's work done on the other. Massive curriculum revision that incorporates in-depth teaching of cancer and other deviations from health is long overdue. Only then can nursing be weaned away from serving the hospital's narrow service activity needs and become ready to meet people's need for help in dealing with their illnesses and their need to sustain and promote their own health.

Note. From "The History of Cancer in the Nursing Curriculum, 1860–1951" (pp. 1–9) by K.R. Nelson in *Cancer Nurses Make it Happen: A Tenth Anniversary History of the Nursing Committee*, 1987, Wallingford, CT: American Cancer Society. Copyright 1987 by American Cancer Society. Excerpted with permission.

TRIBUTES

My years at Teachers College, Columbia University, constituted some of the most memorable experiences of my life. A very, very large part of the reason for this was my introduction to and continued contact with Dr. Katherine R. Nelson. Dr. Nelson was my academic adviser, but she was much more than that. She was an accomplished teacher, an encouraging and knowledgeable guide, and a professional mentor in every sense of the symbol. Katherine was an indefatigable and exemplary support system for those of us fortunate enough to have her as an adviser.

Dr. Nelson's contributions to the nursing profession are legendary. Her commitment to the primary mission of Teachers College (i.e., excellence in education) was most pronounced. Also, her dedication to her students' success and career development was awesome in both scope and practice. Dr. Nelson's nationally recognized service to the community could be seen in her long-standing and highly regarded work in the care of cancer victims. Helping others, especially her involvement in the teaching/learning process, was Katherine's mission in life.

Dr. Nelson was not only a legend but also a leader. My experiences with her may be best summarized with a quotation from the Book of Tao entitled "The Best Leader."

As for the best leaders, the people do not notice their existence. The next best, the people honor and praise. The next, the people fear; and the next, the people hate. If you have no faith, people will have no faith in you, and you must resort to oaths. When the best leader's work is done the people say: "We did it ourselves!"

Joseph R. Proulx, RN, EdD

Professor
University of Maryland
Baltimore, MD

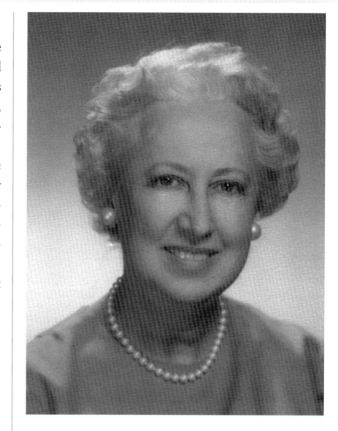

ABOVE
Katherine Nelson

I first contacted Dr. Nelson in 1973 to seek her input on possible directions that we might take to formally organize ourselves as oncology nurses. On the phone, she came across as a gracious lady and a true veteran educator and caregiver. Dr. Nelson reviewed the complete history of the

KATHERINE R. NELSON

founding of the National League of Nursing as an example of the organizational process. I discussed with her the possibility of assembling our group under the umbrella of the American Nurses Association as another alternative. We also discussed how nursing had evolved from the 1940s to the present (1973 at the time), noting that many more resources were available to nurses caring for patients with cancer. We agreed that it wasn't just the lack of available resources that hindered nursing care during the 1940s but the stigma and secrecy associated with the diagnosis of cancer as well. People didn't openly discuss their diagnosis as they do now. Treatments were limited, and pain control was a major issue.

In the early 1970s, the role of nurses in clinical care was still limited. We talked about the emerging role of the clinical nurse specialist in cancer, especially since I just had finished my master's degree and was functioning in this very role. Nurses cared for patients with cancer but weren't really considered part of the care team. We talked about how the perception of nursing needed to change, especially if cancer nurses were to be regarded as partners with physicians in cancer care. Expectations of physicians, patients, and their families (about what nurses could contribute) needed to change.

While some content of my 1973 conversation with Dr. Nelson may appear to be very dated to young nurses today, it is important to recognize that these were very challenging issues for us to deal with during that time. In addition to convincing others about our capabilities and interests in caring for patients with cancer, nurses themselves needed to be encouraged to participate more actively and to enroll in continuing-education programs.

Dr. Nelson's role as a premiere educator was also a major topic in our conversation. She had a clear vision of what it took to prepare advanced practice nurses. She wanted to hear about the graduate oncology-nursing program that I had created at Rush College of Nursing in 1972. We compared notes, so to speak.

It was after this lengthy discussion that I asked her to serve as an advisor to the Oncology Nursing Society. I mentioned that I wasn't sure which direction we ultimately would follow in the process of organizing, but I felt that it was important that we continue to seek substantive input from pioneers like her.

During the next several years, Dr. Nelson continued her supportive approach with all of us. She conveyed to us her very firm belief that regardless of how we chose to organize, we should set very high standards for ourselves. Recall of past events is not perfect by any means, but I truly believe that it was Dr. Nelson who inspired me the most to believe that a nursing organization could strive to combine clinical, educational, and research foci. At the time, nursing organizations tended to focus only on one of these aspects rather than trying to attract nurses who were clinicians, educators, or researchers, bringing them together that they might communicate and learn from each other.

The Oncology Nursing Society went on to do just that, and one of the pioneers to whom we owe a great deal is Dr. Katherine Nelson!

Lisa Begg, DrPH

Chief, Cancer Training Branch
National Cancer Institute
Bethesda, MD

Professional papers and effects of Katherine Nelson are located in the archives at the National Office of the Oncology Nursing Society in Pittsburgh, PA.

EDITH S. WOLF, RN, MA
Leader in Cancer Education for Patients and Nursing Staff

"One of the greatest challenges in cancer nursing is teaching the patient self-management. It is much easier for a nurse to give a nasal feeding or colostomy irrigation than it is to spend time teaching the patient how to do it. However, when the nurse becomes involved in teaching patients self-management . . . the anxiety created by extensive surgery is usually replaced with a sense of satisfaction in the patient's accomplishments."
— Edith S. Wolf

EDITH S. WOLF

SIGNIFICANT CAREER CONTRIBUTIONS

- Only woman and nurse member for five years on the National Professional Education Committee of the American Cancer Society

- Advocated for self-care through patient teaching

- Authored several patient-education booklets

- Helped initiate team nursing and the use of the Kardex System at Memorial Sloan-Kettering Cancer Center

BIOGRAPHICAL INFORMATION

BIRTH AND DEATH

Edith Schweighofer was born on August 11, 1908, in Scranton, PA. She died January 31, 1995, in Waymart, PA.

PARENTS

Edith was one of two children, both daughters, born to Charles M. Schweighofer and Edith Philman Avery. Both of Edith's parents were born and raised in Honesdale, PA, where they later established the family farm. In the later years of their lives, Edith's parents spent the winters with her and her husband, Milton, in New York City and spent the rest of the year at the farm. Edith and Milton retired to the farm from New York and named the property "Hickory Hill."

FAMILY

Edith and her sister, Grace, both attended grammar school in Honesdale's one-room schoolhouse. They always walked to school, even in the deep snows of winter. After graduating from Honesdale High School in 1924, Edith worked for three years as a secretary at the Citizen's Publishing Company. Edith had a lifelong interest in writing and journalism that she never pursued academically, but she did make a substantial contribution to the nursing literature. After her years at the Citizen's Publishing Company, Edith worked for two years as an assistant in the office of an ear, nose, and throat physician. Whether Edith's interest in nursing preceded her work in this position or whether this experience stimulated her entrance to nursing school is not clear. However, within the area of cancer care, she had a special clinical interest in head and neck cancers and performed substantial work in this area.

CAREER PATH

MT. SINAI HOSPITAL

Edith was slightly older than her fellow students at Mt. Sinai Hospital, and, as a senior, she often was called on to serve as charge nurse, especially on the off shifts. These administration aspects of the senior-year curriculum came very naturally to her. Edith viewed Mt. Sinai as an old and highly respected institution, and when she was offered the position of head nurse, she readily accepted. In 1944, she served as assistant supervisor in the outpatient department and also served as a clinical instructor and associate director of the Nursing Education Program. During this time, Edith contracted tuberculosis from a patient and spent a year in the Tuberculosis Sanitorium in Saranac Lake, NY.

While at Mt. Sinai, Edith was active in a number of professional organizations, including the American Nurses Association, the National League for Nursing, the Mt. Sinai Alumnae Association (past president), and the Mt. Sinai Foundation (past president). She also served as director of District #13 of the New York Counties Registered Nurses' Association. Her professional network grew through these organizational affiliations and through her schoolwork at the Teachers College at Columbia University.

Cancer was not Edith's sole professional interest while at Mt. Sinai, although numerous patients with cancer were treated there. A designated cancer unit did not exist at that time, and patients with cancer were dispersed throughout the in- and outpatient units.

Several factors influenced Edith's decision to leave Mt. Sinai after 20 years of service. She recently had completed her bachelor's degree in hospital administration at Columbia University and was eager to put some of her new knowledge to work. She looked at possible opportunities at Mt. Sinai and felt that upward mobility in administration was very limited, because the practice was for those reaching the highest positions to maintain them until retirement.

About this time, she was approached to interview at Memorial Center for Cancer and Allied Diseases, which is now Memorial Sloan-Kettering Cancer Center in New York City. She was very impressed with some of the learning and teaching opportunities that would be open to her. "If you will only come," they said, "your first experience will be a big one. We have 43 women to be trained as nurses' aides." This proved to be her first major assignment.

MEMORIAL CENTER FOR CANCER AND ALLIED DISEASES

Edith assumed the position of Associate Director of Nursing Education at Memorial Center for Cancer and Allied Diseases, where she reported to Thelma Laird, who was Director of Nursing from 1954–1959. Edith was the third person to hold this position, following Katherine Nelson and Margaret Coleman (Asadorian et al., 1984).

During the 20 years Edith was at Memorial Hospital, she reported to three different directors of nursing. These directors oversaw the entire nursing department but also had responsibilities specific to the development of the hospital during their tenure, which had implications for the work of Edith's department. Thelma Laird made organizing orientation for new appointees a priority and developed policies governing the practice of nursing. Affiliations with university programs were instituted, and team nursing was introduced.

When Thelma resigned in 1960 for health reasons, Mary Connolly was appointed as Director of Nursing. Recruitment was a major challenge during Mary's administration, and staffing the evening tour of duty and the new pediatrics unit was difficult. Negative attitudes toward cancer

ATTITUDES

One of the most basic objectives in preparing a nurse to work with patients with cancer is to help her understand and accept, first, the disease itself, and, second, the "aggressive" treatment that may be necessary.

The nurse's attitude is all-important. If she understands and accepts our philosophy in relation to aggressive treatment—extensive surgery or radiation—she can then formulate her own philosophy and acceptance of the disease or its treatment. To build and maintain a positive attitude is not easy, but, if the nurse is thoroughly oriented to all aspects of the disease and its treatment, she is on the way to a beginning practice of the quality of excellence in nursing care.

In our orientation program we try to help nurses develop a positive attitude toward cancer and its treatment. To understand and accept the philosophy that underlies aggressive treatment for an aggressive disease may be difficult, but, if the nurse remembers the moribund child who was brought in, given chemical agents (that seem to make him even more ill), and then, in a few days, is up playing, she learns to build and maintain a positive attitude.

WOLF, 1968, P. 41

EDITH S. WOLF

Common treatments performed during January–June 1968 at Memorial Hospital

- 6,747 cleansing sprays (e.g., mouth, groin, breast, perineum, decubitus)
- 4,447 dressings
- 191 bone marrow aspirations
- 145 thoracenteses
- 129 proctoscopies and sigmoidoscopies
- 57 paracenteses

MYERS, WOLF, & LACHER, 1968

RIGHT
A teaching slide showing a head and neck treatment room nurse spraying and suctioning the oral cavity at the same time.

nursing prevailed. Rotations of nurses to off shifts were instituted, and Edith was in charge of establishing orientation and in-service programs for these shifts. The opening of Sloan House, an apartment building for nurses, was seen as an incentive. In addition, bonuses for nurses in terms of tuition refunds and an expanded in-service training program were emphasized. Each had an impact on the work of Edith's department.

Prior to Mary's retirement, plans were made for the Memorial nurses to take over the staffing of the James Ewing Hospital, a city-run cancer hospital in New York within the Memorial Hospital property. The immediate need for 100 additional registered nurses had obvious implications for the education department. Memorial Hospital increased in scope, and the medical specialty of oncology became more refined. The first coronary-care and special-care units were opened, as well as a neurology unit. All of these initiatives had an impact on Edith's position as an educator.

One of the factors that influenced Edith's decision to assume the position of Associate Director of Nursing Education at Memorial Hospital was the way in which the patients' medical services were organized by site (e.g., bone, breast, bowel). Weekly conferences were held for each service, with a variety of disciplines interacting. Nurses were encouraged to attend and participate in the conferences. Another component of organization by cancer site was the presence of nurse specialists and specialized treatment rooms. This approach had been in place for many years before Edith's arrival and was based on the recognition that numerous special procedures would be performed better under examining room conditions rather than at the bedside. For the approximately 273 beds, six treatment rooms were available. The use of treatment rooms for special procedures and the availability of specially prepared nurses facilitated performing the procedures with increased dignity, efficiency, and comfort for the patients and with greater speed and satisfaction for the physician.

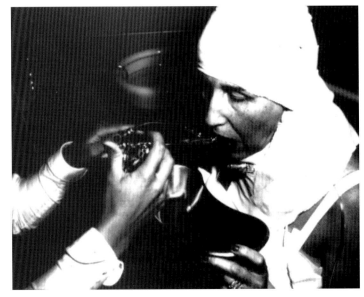

The treatment-room registered nurses received special on-the-job training that included learning to spray cleansing solution on wounds and in the mouth, changing tracheotomy and laryngectomy tubes, dressing wounds, inserting packings, inserting nasal feeding tubes, and teaching patients self-care.

The treatment rooms had assigned staff who required orientation as turnover occurred. In addition, many of the students and nurses in educational programs at Memorial Hospital observed or participated in procedures in one or more of the treatment rooms.

The hospital placed an emphasis on active treatment rather than terminal care. Very aggressive treatment was the norm, especially in surgery and radiation therapy. Without today's vast armamentarium of chemotherapy, the belief was that aggressive surgical approaches offered patients the best hope. Some of the staff had difficulty accepting the extent of the surgery performed. Nurses needed assistance with both the intensive physical care required by patients and how to deal with the psychosocial aspects of treatment and disease.

During Edith's 20-year tenure at Memorial Hospital, she saw dramatic changes in every arena. Her role was multifaceted, and, in an institution as large and complex as Memorial Hospital, separating the activities she led from those in which she had active collaboration was difficult. The breadth of the role of nursing during those years and just how much nurses were able to accomplish is more impressive than just who did what. Edith's job description had included functions in the categories of planning and organization, reporting, budgeting, teaching, evaluation, and study and research (Memorial Hospital for Cancer and Allied Diseases, Division of Nursing, 1967). Twenty-six functions were delineated within the category of planning and organization; examples include

- Reviews current methods of treatment for procedure change within the center
- Secures information on current practices from authoritative sources
- Secures information from other community institutions and agencies so that "common practice" is known
- Schedules in-service programs and secures classrooms, speakers, films, and projectionist for day, evening, and night meetings
- Coordinates and plans with Teachers' College instructors each semester fieldwork experiences for leadership and cancer nursing students; cooperates and plans with individual universities, colleges, and hospitals for extended visits and independent studies by nurses; counsels and guides nurses in all clinical experiences
- Plans and arranges field trips for 500–1,000 nursing students and individual nurses each year, domestic and foreign, for visiting the center, thereby promoting the development of cancer nursing throughout the world

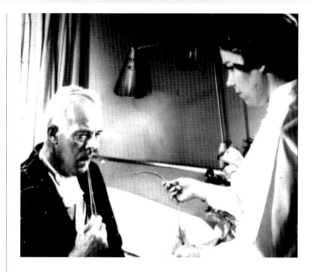

ABOVE
A teaching slide showing the use of a Y tube, which enables the catheter used to suction the tracheotomy or laryngectomy tube and the metal suction tip used to suction the mouth to use the same trap bottle and source of suction

EDITH S. WOLF

- Participates in cancer nursing programs throughout the United States by teaching in universities as well as joining one-day meetings and panel discussions at the national, state, and district levels, thus promoting nurse recruitment and public relationship
- Counsels and guides nurses who are attending college and records and signs tuition refunds
- Arranges for scholarship funds and their awarding
- Arranges for all teas, flowers, and rooms
- Plans and arranges exhibits to be shown at national nursing conventions.

One function states, "Tries to provide for development of an environment which fosters a productive teaching-learning situation." The statement is followed parenthetically with the sentence, "This has been impossible because of lack of *adequate* classrooms; also the *absolute* lack of controlled room temperature." The functions are interesting to consider as a reflection of the scope of work and how it was to be accomplished. Participating in nursing programs throughout the United States and reviewing current practice seem vast in terms of responsibility, given the lack of resource materials and organizations at the time. Arranging for teas and flowers is a function not likely to be found in a similar position description today. From the job description, archival materials, and Edith's own notes, three primary role functions are apparent: in-service education, patient education, and nursing recruitment.

In-service education: Initially, training nurses' aides (and later overseeing that program), orienting nurses new to the setting, and promoting the continuing education of nurses already in practice were major components of the in-service role. Valuable insight into the approaches for meeting the emotional needs of nurses working in this setting are found in Edith's writings, especially in two *Nursing Outlook* papers, "Where Hope Comes First" (1964) and "Nurse Clinician in a Specialty Hospital" (1968). It was important for each level of nursing to emphasize the "challenge of helping the patient to become self-sufficient and independent, to lift his morale and give him a sense of security. Most important, we cultivate an attitude of hope toward the disease and its treatment" (Wolf, 1964, p. 52). Patients often were told that they had a "tumor," and a reliable family member was given further information. Whether to tell the patient more was under discussion at many centers at that time. In Edith's experience, patients often did not ask for more information, and part of the hospital's philosophy at that time was to keep hope alive. Edith found that sometimes patients were told more than they actually wanted to know at a particular time. Edith felt it often was the physician's need to tell the patient that was being met and not the patient's need to know. Edith noted two areas of conviction—patients must be told everything or they must be told nothing. "This is somewhat surprising when one reflects that the nurse in caring for patients with other diseases accepts and appears satisfied with what the doctor tells the patient and performs accordingly. Why then must every diagnostic detail be forced on the cancer patient?" (Wolf, 1964, p. 52).

The implementation of team nursing as a model of practice and the use of the nursing Kardex System for planning patient care and recording aspects of the patient's treatment plan began at Memorial Hospital in the 1950s. When Thelma Laird became director of nursing, she felt that the concept of team nursing being promoted by Eleanor Lambertson at Teachers College, Columbia University, might fit well with the care delivery needs at Memorial Hospital. Team nursing faculty assigned the care of a group of patients to a group of caregivers, both professional and support personnel. A registered nurse usually assumed the role of team leader and divided the care of the patients according to their needs and the skills of the team members. Usually, one nurse gave the medications and another undertook treatment. Personal care for the patient and simple treatments, such as ambulating and range of motion exercises, were the responsibilities of a team member, frequently a nurse's aide. With Eleanor's assistance, a program was developed to help the Division of Nursing make the transition to team nursing. Hour-long workshops were offered on each unit by Columbia professor Edna Danielson. The nurses and nurses' aides needed orientation to team nursing. The program was not easily accepted, and many head nurses saw this practice model as a threat to their power. The model remained in place for 20 years, with its weaknesses—fragmentation of care, shared responsibility and accountability, and uneven work distribution—addressed on an ongoing basis.

BELOW
A team nursing conference in which the Kardex System is being used to review patient-care plans. The team shown here includes two registered nurses and two nurses' aides, modeled on the system promoted by Eleanor Lambertson.

In addition to the general in-service programming, staff members were invited to take part in many of the films and lecture programs given to participants of the various internships and university programs, which offered a wide variety of topics. The schedule for the June 1950 grouping of 16 undergraduate students attending the four- or six-week New York University program provided approximately three hours a day of physician lectures. Topics included science and research in cancer, skin and

EDITH S. WOLF

Perhaps it is surprising that, in a cancer specialty hospital, our nursing staff is comprised of young, eager, and enthusiastic nurses. They are nurses who possess a positive attitude toward cancer and its treatment; are prepared to work with and accept the challenge of meeting any type of emergency; have the ability and patience to teach self-management to patients with disfigurement or change in bodily function; and are able to help patients return to society. Patients can do this without creating a major change in their way of life and can become active citizens once again. In fact, patients often return to their old jobs.

The atmosphere in which the nurses work is pleasant, cheerful, and optimistic. It creates a climate in which the patient can be relaxed, cheerful, and hopeful. Also, it may come as a surprise that these nurses are not threatened by, nor do they resign because of, the disease and its treatment. They resign for the usual reasons—marriage, pregnancy, or the lure of faraway places.

WOLF, 1968, P. 42

mixed tumors, head and neck tumors, breast tumors, childhood tumors, x-ray therapy, electrolyte balances, and radioactive isotopes (Memorial Hospital for Cancer and Allied Diseases, Division of Nursing, 1950). A 1969 semiannual Nursing Education Department report (Wolf, 1969, pp. 1–4) indicated that the following programs were active:

- Baccalaureate students from Teachers College—Leadership field experience was provided for 10 students in the spring and for 21 students in the summer session.
- Masters' students from Teachers College—Four students of Dr. Katherine Nelson undertook independent studies in the spring semester and 15 participated in the summer session.
- Doctoral student from Teachers College—Shirley Graffam used the hospital as one of five institutions for her dissertation work.
- New York University—A three-week workshop was held with 21 students attending from various areas of the country. Planning was completed with instructors from New York University and Memorial Hospital.
- Internship program—Seventeen students arrived from foreign countries for the spring semester, making a total of 43 nurses in the Ewing Hospital program, which was coordinated by Norma Owens, nursing professor at New York University.
- New York Hospital (Cornell)—Two groups of eight students came two days a week to the outpatient department for clinical experience during the spring semester.
- Orientation—New staff nurses attended one week of classes. One hundred and twenty-eight nurses attended 12 cycles of classes.
- Health physics—Releasing nurses from duty for a 20-hour course continued to be a problem. Two courses were given in this time period, with six nurses in the first group and seven in the second group.
- Visitors—In addition to the students from the various university programs, people from seven states and two countries made 425 visits to the hospital for varying lengths of time and purposes.

This report gives an idea of the variety of programs under way at that time. During the course of Edith's career, Memorial Hospital opened its doors in numerous other situations to provide clinical experiences with cancer to a variety of nurses and students. Many diploma programs from across the city regularly used Memorial Hospital for a clinical experience site. Although these programs brought their own field instructor, the student experiences had to be coordinated and unit placement organized.

Patient education: Of all her accomplishments, Edith felt the most pride in her work in patient teaching. This area always presented a challenge, and she and her colleagues looked for ways to better meet the needs of the patients. Materials were not readily available, and even ACS had few materials on patient care. To meet these needs, Memorial Hospital's nurses developed teaching books to aid both nurses and patients. Two booklets were primarily for nurses: *A Handbook on Radiation for Nurses* and a *Nurse Reference Manual*. Three patient-education booklets (*A Handbook of Nursing Care for Head and Neck Patients*, *Home Care for the Urological Patient*, and *Rehabilitation of the Colostomy Patient*) were developed, printed, and sold through the In-Service Department. The head and neck booklet was in constant demand and was sold to hospitals around the United States.

During much of Edith's tenure at Memorial Hospital, patient-teaching sessions were held each Tuesday and Thursday morning. The focus of these particular classes was rehabilitation, although different classes were available for patients on the different disease-site units.

MEMORIAL HOSPITAL FOR CANCER AND ALLIED DISEASES
TREATMENT UNIT
OF
MEMORIAL SLOAN-KETTERING CANCER CENTER

A HANDBOOK OF

NURSING CARE FOR HEAD AND NECK PATIENTS

THE DEPARTMENT OF NURSING

12th PRINTING, 1972

LEFT
Of all of her accomplishments, Edith was most proud of this patient teaching booklet, shown here in its 12th printing in 1972.

The rehabilitation classes met two needs—the patients themselves obviously benefited from the information shared, and nurse visitors frequently requested the opportunity to observe. In the report cited earlier, Edith recorded that 223 patients attended classes between January and August 1969, and 401 visitors observed the rehabilitation class (Wolf, 1969).

Another class, held two mornings a week, was the arm exercise class for the patients with breast cancer. Originally, a piano player, who was later replaced by a record player, came to the sixth floor solarium to provide music for the patients. The content of the class expanded to include nutrition, hand and arm care, and other nursing care components. The In-Service Department organized the classes, with nurses rotating to lead the classes. Later, social work services were added to the classes.

Nursing recruitment: The recruitment of qualified nurses to work at Memorial Hospital appeared to be an ongoing effort. Cancer continued to be a difficult area for recruitment, and competition among the New York City hospitals for experienced staff was intense. Nurses in lead-

EDITH S. WOLF

BELOW
Nurses in leadership positions were encouraged to participate in professional seminars to enhance the visibility of Memorial Hospital for Cancer and Allied Diseases. Taken at a 1958 Cancer Conference, "Changing Times," at St. John's University, this photograph shows, from left to right, Edith Wolf, Associate Director of Nursing Education, Memorial Hospital for Cancer and Allied Diseases; Mary Mullen, Director of Nursing, Kings County Hospital Center, Brooklyn, NY; Bosse B. Randle, Director of Nursing, Nassau County Department of Health; and Mary A. Miller, Assistant Director and Consultant for Inservice Education, National League for Nursing.

ership roles such as Edith's were encouraged to be active in outside organizations, to accept speaking engagements, and to publish with the intent of increasing the visibility of Memorial Hospital.

Edith was very active with ACS and gave speeches across the United States. She worked closely with three women who had held the title of National Nursing Consultant of ACS—Marjorie Schlotterbeck, Clare Richmond, and Virginia Barckley. Edith enjoyed these opportunities and had great admiration for the work these nurses accomplished in bringing knowledge and support to nurses across the country. She also was a member of the committee that produced the first ACS *Source Book for Nurses.* "You really had to admire what the ACS did for nurses in the community," said Edith in a videotaped interview. "Whether the need was in Portland, Oregon, or Boise, Idaho, the ACS had one of their nurses ready to try and meet those needs." She expressed appreciation at the opportunities that came to her through this work and valued the friendships formed through this professional network. "They talk about experts being people coming from out of town and bringing slides," she said laughingly. She developed an extensive set of slides and was prepared to talk about a variety of subjects—not just the content of her lecture—and she was prepared to answer any question that might come from the audience. Edith related that most of ACS's speakers could discuss breast cancer as well as head and neck cancer or ostomies. Travel expenses usually were covered, but an honorarium did not exist until Edith's last lecture, for which she was given

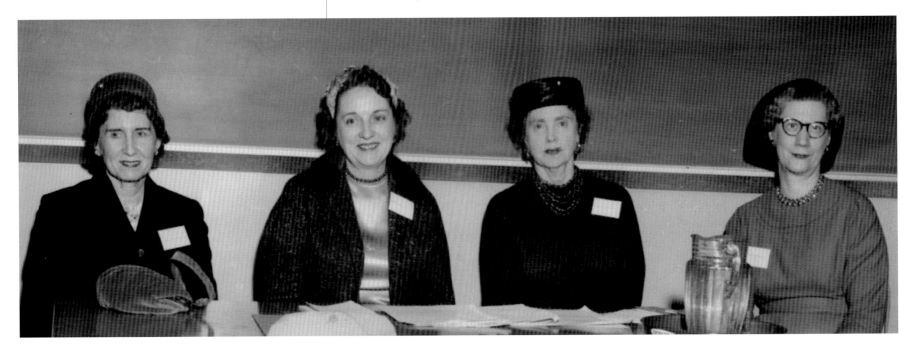

$100. One interesting trip took her on an eight-day jaunt to New Hampshire, where she was in a different location each day giving a different lecture. Another year, she addressed the American Nurses Association in Florida, and another opportunity took her to New Mexico to give a three-week course.

Visibility also was extended through recruitment booths at local and national meetings. During the 1950s and 1960s, recruitment efforts officially were the responsibility of the Assistant Director of Nursing Service, a position held by Veronica Morris Hanlon and later by Delia Brown. In-Service Department staff and other assistant directors regularly helped in these efforts, or, as Edith phrased it, "It was kind of dumped on In-Service." Edith believed that New York City itself was a pull for many nurses, but they needed to be convinced that they wanted to work in cancer and that they could live safely in the city. When the Sloan House was built, the beautiful 18-story apartment building was a good recruitment tool. In addition to providing affordable housing, classroom space was available on the first floor that was used for lectures and social activities. Recruiters looked for certain qualities in the nurses they talked with, such as being able to support the concept of hope while providing good nursing care.

Edith told of an interesting recruitment effort undertaken when the Memorial Hospital nursing staff had to provide staffing for the Ewing Hospital. Recruitment was extremely difficult, and the staff was uncertain of how they would find the needed nurses. A member of the hospital's board of directors knew Argentina's president, Juan Peron. Arrangements were made for the Director of Nursing to travel to Argentina and meet with Juan and Evita Peron in a recruitment effort. Thirteen nurses came to the United States to begin their work at Memorial Hospital. Only one of these nurses was fluent in English, but all of them had to be oriented to the city as well as to the hospital and its procedures. A Spanish-speaking person was assigned to help them, and these nurses attended separate classes until their language difficulties could be addressed. Another recruitment effort brought nurses from the Scandinavian countries. Although

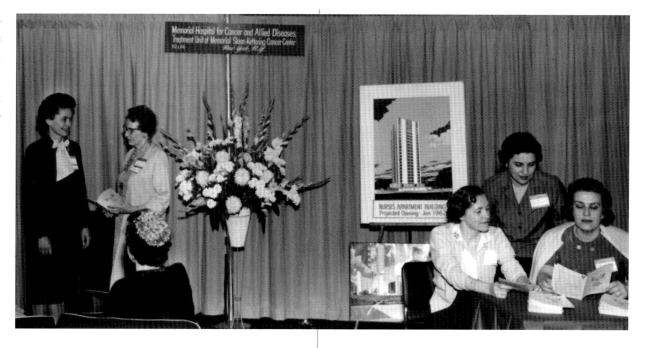

ABOVE
The recruitment booth for Memorial Hospital for Cancer and Allied Diseases at the National League for Nursing Convention, Cleveland, OH, 1961. This display featured opportunities in radiation therapy and showed the architect's rendering of the planned Sloan Building, apartments for nurses. Edith Wolf is second from the left.

EDITH S. WOLF

BELOW

BELOW
As President of the Wayne County Unit of the American Cancer Society (ACS), Edith Wolf is shown here at the Annual Pennsylvania State ACS Convention, Carlisle, PA, March 31, 1978. Shown from left to right are Chuck Naginey, Crusade Chairman, Pennsylvania Division; Nancy Martene, Miss Hope Wayne County, PA; Edith Wolf; and Laverne Thornton, Vice President of the Wayne County ACS Unit.

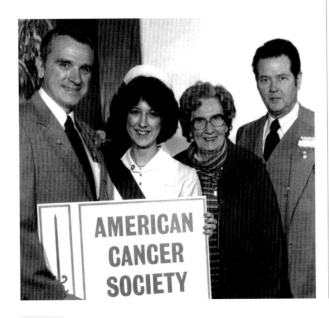

these nurses spoke English fluently, they posed different challenges in orientation. Not one of them had ever seen an adjustable bed.

RETIREMENT

Edith retired from Memorial Hospital in 1969, after almost 20 years of devoted service. In 1972, she was diagnosed with breast cancer and returned to Memorial Hospital for treatment. Her diagnosis and surgery occurred at about the same time as that of Happy Rockefeller. Dr. Jerome Urban treated both women.

Edith and her husband, Milton, continued to be actively involved in volunteer activities. Edith became active with the Wayne County Unit of ACS and continued to do a fair amount of local travel and lecturing. She also organized a number of professional education activities and served as unit president for three years. She continued her nursing involvement through promoting the ACS "Nurse of Hope" program. Edith never seemed to get used to the idea that her vast experience was highly respected in her community and that people remained interested in her views on cancer. She expressed wonder that, "At 80, I was called and asked to speak to the local Rotary Club."

Edith and her husband also became active with the American Red Cross. Although her local activities were new, her affiliation with the American Red Cross was long standing, having begun when she graduated from nursing school. In 1971, Edith fulfilled a long-time dream and traveled to Switzerland to visit the world headquarters of the Red Cross. Locally, she worked with the blood mobile, taking medical histories of the donors. Milton served as Regional Director of the Wilkes-Barre blood bank and was honored for more than 50 years of service. Edith said that it felt natural for her to share this work with her husband. She had seen blood used in conjunction with cancer treatment for so many years that it seemed an appropriate extension of her interests to help to see that the supply was kept available.

Retirement also allowed Edith to become active in other community activities, such as in the Cold Spring-Rileyville Presbyterian Church. With many family members living in close proximity, Edith and Milton were able to keep in close touch with nieces and nephews and their children.

In 1984, Milton died. Edith's niece, Ann Curtis, said that Edith began to "go downhill" after her husband's death. In July of 1994, Edith suffered a stroke, and Ann was no longer able to provide the care that Edith needed. Edith entered a nursing home but was unhappy there and wanted to be "closer to home." She moved to the Wayne Woodlands Manor in Waymart, PA. She died on January 31, 1995, and was buried in East Dyberry Cemetery. She requested that the Honesdale farm be kept in the family. At this time, her grandniece and family are still living there.

SUMMARY

Edith Wolf had a very full career—40 years of nursing service in two facilities. She made lasting contributions at Memorial Sloan-Kettering Cancer Center and Mt. Sinai Hospital of New York.

As one reads about Edith's work and her professional network, she obviously has influenced many nurses new to the field of cancer nursing. She was active in cancer at a time when changes were constant, and she had daily dialogue with the outstanding clinicians at Memorial Hospital, one of the most prestigious centers in the country. Edith was closely affiliated with pioneers in nursing at the Teachers College at Columbia University, such as Dorothy Gordon, Martha Rogers, and Eleanor Lambertson. She also traveled regularly with Marge Schlotterbeck and Virginia Barckley. Edith was one of many outstanding nurses at Memorial Hospital, but her dedication seems representative of the contributions made by nurses in cancer centers during the formative years of cancer nursing as a speciality.

REFERENCES

Asadorian, M., Brown, M.H., Powers, A., Sheehan, M., Studva, K., Sullivan, K., & Wollnik, L. (Eds.). (1984). *A century of oncology nursing 1884–1984*. New York: Memorial Sloan-Kettering Cancer Center.

Memorial Hospital for Cancer and Allied Diseases, Division of Nursing. (1950, June). *Schedule for oncology nurse course*. Unpublished schedule.

Memorial Hospital for Cancer and Allied Diseases, Division of Nursing. (1967). *Position title: Associate director, nursing education*. Unpublished position description.

Myers, E.K., Wolf, E.S., & Lacher, M.J. (1968). *Nurse specialists and specialized treatment rooms improve patient care*. Unpublished manuscript, Memorial Hospital for Cancer and Allied Diseases, New York.

Wolf, E.S. (1964). Where hope comes first. *Nursing Outlook, 12*(4), 52–54.

Wolf, E.S. (1968). Nurse clinician in a specialty hospital. *Nursing Outlook, 16*(6), 40–42.

Wolf, E.S. (1969). *Nursing education report, January 1969–August 1969*. Unpublished report, Memorial Hospital for Cancer and Allied Diseases, Division of Nursing.

Wolf, Edith, interview by Susan Baird, 1987.

EDITH S. WOLF

SELECTED WRITINGS

NURSING CARE OF THE PATIENT WITH BREAST CANCER (1968)

The Nurse's Role in Setting the Climate for the Patient With Breast Cancer

Summary

Patient teaching is one of the most important and challenging functions of the nurse. Regardless of where the nurse works she should be alert and prepared to accept the challenge so that no patient is ever heard to say "I had to learn for myself."

All women including nurses should be encouraged to practice breast self-examination a few days after the menstrual period and to continue the practice after the menopause.

One of the most difficult tasks in nursing is to develop a positive attitude toward cancer as a disease and toward the aggressive treatment which may be necessary. Once this is accomplished, the nurse can then begin to help the patient who is fearful, anxious, and depressed.

Following surgery the important function of the nurse is to assist the patient to early rehabilitation both psychologic and physical, by teaching her exercises, proper posture, knowledge of prostheses, and grooming.

Note. From "Nursing Care of the Patient With Breast Cancer," by E.S. Wolf, 1968, *Nursing Clinics of North America*, 2(4), pp. 587–598. Copyright 1968 by W.B. Saunders Company. Excerpted with permission.

NURSE CLINICIAN IN A SPECIALTY HOSPITAL (1968)

In a specialty hospital—in this case for cancer—nurses can develop an optimistic, compassionate attitude after effective orientation and continuing in-service education.

Most nurses employed for the first time in a specialty hospital need orientation—to the particular techniques, the setting, and, most particularly, the patients they will be caring for. Cancer, like neurology, cardiac surgery, and psychiatry, to name a few, is no exception. There is much more to cancer nursing than new techniques.

I will discuss here the clinical specialist or nurse clinician in terms of the nurse working with patients with cancer in a specialty hospital. These nurses work all tours of duty, as well as weekends, and they work in a milieu which is necessarily fraught with emotion and danger at all times, whether treatment is surgery, radiation therapy, or chemotherapy. In this climate, the nurse performs in a highly skilled, compassionate manner; she must also be technically competent. She is not required to have previous specialty experience or education, since we are able to instruct, prepare, and support the nurse in this clinical specialty, as well as the aide who will assist her.

Teaching Patient Self-Management

Nurses are often frustrated and may suffer traumatic experience unless they understand that they cannot project themselves into the patient's position. They are not the patients with cancer, suffering pain and disruption of life; they must remember that the patient has come asking for help—it is he who made the choice. If the answer for him is mutilating facial surgery, then the nurse must reassure him and teach him about the many procedures that will follow surgery, procedures that will help him become a confident, secure person, reliant in his own self-management.

The patient skilled in self-management is always proud to demonstrate his proficiency to others. His personal satisfaction in teaching other patients is always a challenge to the specialty bedside nurse. Nurses working with other aggressive types of treatment, such as open-heart surgery, hyperbaric oxygenation therapy, organ transplants, and the like, also have to build and maintain positive attitudes, else they would be overwhelmed with negative feelings.

A nurse with a positive attitude can approach her patient with knowledge and self-confidence that will inspire him with confidence and encourage him in his acceptance of treatment. Her attitude greatly affects the patient's reaction toward both his disease and his outlook for the future.

Inservice

By means of leadership or team nursing, the professional nurse relates closely to the nursing aide in the clinical situation and helps the aide to understand and work with patients without stress or fear. As in a general hospital, we are concerned with monitors, the Brewer system of giving medications, and complicated inhalation therapy machines. This calls for a great deal of inservice training constantly available. Our services are not divided into medical, surgical, pediatrics, and so on, but anatomically: head and neck, breast, bone, thoracic, gastric, and mixed tumor, for example. Each service holds a weekly doctor's conference, where patients and their specific problems are discussed. As part of inservice, nurses are urged to attend the conferences as often as possible. Specific inservice education on specialty subjects are held frequently on all tours of duty. If the speaker is available only during the day, we tape the lecture so that the evening and night staffs may hear him, either in groups or alone, by taking the tape recorder from one floor to another in the small hours—depending on the work load.

Nursing aides

The nursing aide orientation lasts for three weeks and includes classes and clinical practice; then the aide is assigned to nursing service to work with the professional nurse as a member of the team.

EDITH S. WOLF

Research

In research areas, such as the "life island," nurses are oriented to the clinical unit and taught specifics related to this kind of nursing care. The life island isolator is used for patients with adult leukemia and others with different types of tumors who are receiving chemotherapy and are under close study in cooperation with the National Cancer Institute at the Clinical Center, National Institutes of Health, Bethesda, Maryland.

The isolator is used for those patients with leukemia whose resistance to infection is lowered by their disease, and where control of infection from the environment is vital. Placing the patient in the "sterile bubble" controls all factors involved in daily living.

In general, the nurse is responsible for the preparation and maintenance of reverse isolation. The nurses rotate shifts and work closely with the doctors, dietitians, and others. They are highly skilled and technically competent, true. But they are also gentle and compassionate nurses who continuously strive to give quality nursing care.

Note. From "Nurse Clinician in a Specialty Hospital," by E.S. Wolf, 1968, *Nursing Outlook, 16*(6), pp. 40–42. Copyright 1968 by Mosby Inc. Excerpted with permission.

TRIBUTE

Almost a half century has elapsed since I first met Edith Wolf when she was Associate Director of Nursing Education at Memorial Hospital for Cancer and Allied Diseases, now known as Memorial Sloan-Kettering Cancer Center. Not long after I met her, I realized that I was working with a true professional whose vision and mission were to advance the practice of cancer nursing. Her ability to articulate the contributions nurses make to the care of patients with cancer placed Edith as a leading forerunner of the Oncology Nursing Society.

Although history has documented her contributions at the national level, Edith was equally impressive in the workplace. She took a personal interest in the education and preparation of bedside nurses, which, in the era of diploma school education, was an uphill battle. Her persistence and concern for staff who demonstrated an interest in increasing their knowledge of cancer nursing and acquiring credentials enabled her to gain access for them to hospital-based programs and local universities. Because of Edith's recommendations, tuition reimbursement became a reality before it became an institutional policy. This same level of interest was extended to ancillary personnel. It was very rewarding to welcome back nursing assistants whom she mentored to complete high school and enroll in an LPN program.

Edith was quick to recognize staff potential for advancement in education and administrative roles. Through her contacts with the American Cancer Society, she traveled nationwide to lecture and participate in panel discussions, identifying opportunities for staff to share their knowledge and develop their skills in public speaking. She was a true professional nurse. During a time when nurses in oncology were not considered part of a specialized area of care but simply considered hospital staff members, Edith served as a role model in her total commitment to cancer nursing as a specialty. My debt to Edith is that she provided exposure for me to advance in a leadership role and showed me how to mentor nurses for whom I later provided guidance.

Mary H. Brown, RN, MA
Former Director of Nursing Practice
Memorial Sloan-Kettering Cancer Center
New York, NY

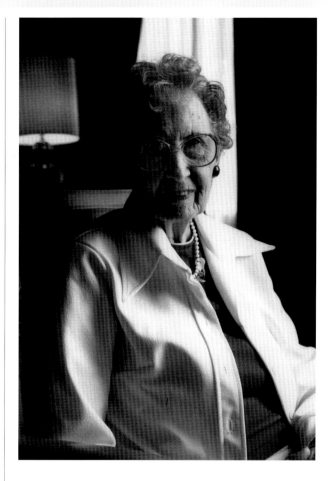

ABOVE
Edith Wolf

Professional papers and effects of Edith Wolf are located in the archives at the National Office of the Oncology Nursing Society in Pittsburgh, PA.

DORIS DILLER, RN, MA
Leader in Surgical Cancer Nursing and Education

"The patient wants empathy, not sympathy. He wants the nurse to be genuinely interested in him and he wishes to be made to feel that she is treating him as she would like herself to be treated. Patients do not want to be pitied."

— *Doris Diller*

DORIS DILLER

SIGNIFICANT CAREER CONTRIBUTIONS

- Recipient of National Cancer Institute (NCI) grants to study cancer knowledge among students in 91 schools of nursing

- Project Director of an NCI grant to integrate cancer nursing into the baccalaureate curriculum

- Coauthor with Edward S. Stafford of *Textbook of Surgery for Nurses* (1947) with two successive editions, *A Textbook of Surgery for Nurses* (1954) and *Surgery and Surgical Nursing* (1958).

RIGHT
Diller children
Doris and Weldon

BIOGRAPHICAL INFORMATION

BIRTH

Doris Leona Diller was born on March 20, 1909, in Columbus Grove, OH.

PARENTS

Doris Diller was one of two children and the only daughter of John Allen and Amelia Reichenbach Diller, who both were born and raised in western Ohio. John left school after eighth grade, but he had a firm conviction that a good education was essential for a secure future. He was a farmer who raised thoroughbred cattle, a special and expensive strain that came from Switzerland to Canada. In 1919, Doris' father sold his herd on the advice of his father, who predicted a crash in the farm market. This advice proved sage, because John was able to sell the herd and the farm at a very good price before the fall, after which many other farmers lost all they owned.

FAMILY

In 1919, John moved his family to Pandora, OH, where they lived on the edge of town so that the family could keep a cow. Doris recalls that she and her brother were allowed to drink milk only from their own cow because bovine tuberculosis was pandemic, and Ohio did not yet require pasteurization of the milk supply or testing of the animals. Doris' mother had a grade-school education and maintained the household.

At age four, Doris was riding with her mother in their wagon when the horse bolted, apparently frightened by a passing automobile. Her mother was thrown from the wagon, and Doris was left to gather the reins and try to control the horse. Amelia received extensive internal injuries requiring surgery. Afterward, she was cared for at home by a series of nurses who lived with the family and cared for the children as well. The children came

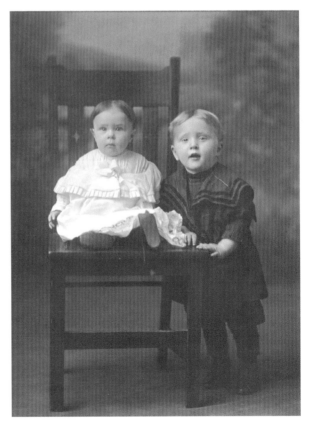

to love these nurses, and Doris became especially close to one of them, Mary Slusser. Doris decided that she too would be a nurse, just as good and kind as Mary, whom she described as "the most wonderful person." These nurses also may have influenced her brother, Weldon, who later became a country doctor. Eventually, Doris' mother recovered completely from her injuries and lived to be 98 years old.

Doris first went to school at the age of five, when she accompanied Weldon to the town's one-room schoolhouse for a visit. The teacher sent home a note saying that although Doris was young to start first grade, she might just as well start coming to school every day because she obviously was ready to start learning. Doris attended the one-room schoolhouse until the family's move to Pandora, a Swiss Mennonite community of approximately 400 people, when she was in sixth grade. A mix of languages was spoken in the area—English, German, and Swiss—and Doris and her brother knew some of each. She recalled that they often had to decide what language they were going to use while they played.

As a result of their parents' strong belief in education, Weldon went off to Ohio State University to study entomology and later medicine. John frequently expressed his beliefs that "Children belong in school" and "children need an education." Doris attended Bluffton College, a Mennonite school approximately six miles from her home. She lived in the dormitory during the week and traveled home on weekends. Doris majored in biology and carried a heavy course load, always taking 18 credits. For her final summer semester, Doris studied economics at DePaul University in Chicago. She said this was the most difficult work she ever undertook. It was the summer of 1929 and the economics professor was forecasting the market crash that came only months later.

When asked why she did not begin to study nursing right away, Doris stated two reasons. First, her father was not really in favor of her going into nursing. "He thought it was very hard work." The second reason was that many schools required that entering students be at least 20 years of age, and Doris had graduated from high school at 17. "They wanted some of the growing up to have taken place before students started in nursing," she said. When her father realized that Doris still was intent on going into nursing, he insisted that she go to the best possible school available. A second cousin, Martha Diller, had graduated from The Johns Hopkins Hospital School of Nursing in 1916, and another Pandora girl had gone there as well, which helped in the decision of what school she would attend.

In September 1929, Doris boarded a train to Baltimore to travel to nursing school. On the way, she stopped overnight in Washington, DC, to visit the museums her father thought she should see. About half of the entering class of 76 people were college graduates, a picture that changed rapidly among diploma programs in the years to come. Within six months, the class was down to about half

DORIS DILLER

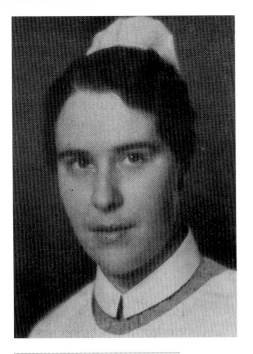

ABOVE
Doris Diller, graduation
photograph of 1932

Photo courtesy of The Johns Hopkins Hospital

of its original number. "Those [who] did not like it or could not do it found out fairly quickly and left," Doris said. Students lived in a residence connected to the hospital. Elsie Lawler, whose name is familiar to nursing historians, was the director of the school. Most of the classes were held in an amphitheater-style room that previously had been an operating theater. As was usual in the clinical curriculum, students proceeded on a regular rotation through various clinical assignments. Doris, however, "got lost in Marburg," as she put it. Marburg was the pavilion for private patients in this 1,200-bed hospital, where clinic and private patients were in separate buildings. For eight months, she was the only student on the unit and drew the worst assignments, working from 7–9 am, 4–6 pm, and 7–11 pm. The units were crowded with patients who probably would have been cared for at home by nurses around the clock were it not for the desperate economics of the Depression.

Doris got "found" again, in terms of her student clinical rotations, when she got sick. She was diagnosed with pneumococcal pneumonia and meningitis and was put into isolation. Treatment included morphine to slow her heart and retention enemas to administer fluids. She was sent home to recover over the next nine weeks and then returned to school to a new clinical assignment.

Doris described herself as a "lazy" student. She found that much of the course work repeated content that she already had learned at Bluffton College. When the material was new to her, she learned rapidly, but when it was material she knew, she figured she could pass the State Board Examinations for Licensure without putting in too much effort. When Doris actually "sat for the boards," she turned in her papers without finishing the last section of questions, which today she finds difficult to acknowledge. At the time, she felt she had answered enough questions to achieve a passing score, and it did not occur to her that the actual score might matter in the future. She knew she would pass and that was enough.

Doris never married. "Didn't have time," she said. She considered marriage and remembers a time, when she was about 37, that she gave serious thought to whether she wanted to be married. "I didn't want to be poor," is another reason Doris gave for not marrying. The Depression was a hard time for young people, and Doris recalled that many of her friends in new marriages found it difficult to obtain work and make ends meet. Doris has maintained close relationships with her brother's family, his daughters, and their children and grandchildren.

CAREER PATH

THE JOHNS HOPKINS HOSPITAL

Many diploma school graduates at this time worked primarily in homes as private duty nurses. Doris, however, decided to work as a staff nurse at the hospital's Wilmer Eye Institute, an ophthalmologic facility renowned for its outstanding physicians and advanced procedures. Many well-known people came to the institute for care. Doris' most famous patient was J.P. Morgan. He asked her where she was from, and when she replied that she was from Bluffton, he said, "Why that was where John Dillinger shot up the town." She was surprised that he had even heard of Bluffton. As a graduate nurse, Doris initially lived in a nursing residence above the hospital's post office but later was given a $20 per month allowance to live on her own outside of the hospital.

After three years at Wilmer, Doris decided that she wanted to give private duty nursing a try. She was not feeling "quite right" and thought the change might be good. She turned out to have rheumatic fever, which was a very serious disease at the time. For three-and-a-half months, she was on bed rest at the hospital, which was located in her familiar student territory. After discharge, she went home to recover, "broke" and unable to work. After sufficient recovery, her doctor allowed her to go back to work on a cycle of working for three months and then taking a month off to rest. Doris looks back on this private duty experience with great affection. She had terribly hard cases and learned a lot. She met many other nurses who were doing this type of work, and she felt a tremendous admiration for their skills and dedication.

In 1941, it was obvious that war was approaching, and Doris was asked to help to train nursing aides at a program initiated by The Johns Hopkins Hospital. The purpose of the program was to secure an adequate patient-care staff, as many of the hospital's medical and nursing staff were preparing to go overseas to form medical units. Some senior nursing students even spent their final year overseas as part of the hospital's response to the need during the war, but Doris knew she would never be approved for war duty because of the residual heart murmur from her bout with rheumatic fever. Instead, she took on the task of training the aides, spending half her time teaching and the other half in the hospital front office. She wrote letters, solved problems, and performed other administrative tasks far removed from patient care, and she hated it. Anna D. Wolf, another renowned Hopkins nursing leader, was the administrator and knew that Doris hated her front-office work. She assigned Doris to the Halsted Building (named after Dr. William Halsted of Halsted hemostat, Halsted suture, and Halsted radical mastectomy fame), the surgical unit of Johns Hopkins, to assume the dual position of Senior Instructor and Nursing Supervisor.

During the next 11 years in the Halsted unit, Doris achieved recognized expertise in surgical nursing. She became an instructor even though she had no formal introduction to teaching. War efforts had swelled the size of the nursing school classes to 170 students entering twice a year. Providing sufficient procedure demonstrations to this number of students proved challenging. Doris solved the problem by demonstrating procedures in an auditorium. She demonstrated colostomy irrigations, dressing changes, and other surgical procedures to the large number of students by taking the patient to the auditorium where she could show each procedure step by step, provid-

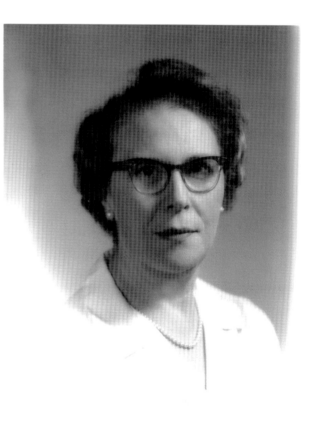

ing patient teaching and support as she went. Doris emphasized to students to "always ask why" and told them that such questioning would always serve them well in practice and in research.

During this time, Doris also assisted with medical student instruction by accompanying all patients to teaching rounds. The role of the nurse was to attend to the patient, protect the patient's privacy and dignity, and make sure that the patient's needs were met during the teaching rounds. In sitting through all of these medical lectures, Doris became a true expert in surgical care. She repeated the surgical course 44 times. She worked closely with Dr. Alfred Blalock (of the famous Blalock-Hanlon palliative operation for transposition of the great vessels and the Blalock-Taussig palliative cardiac shunt for tetralogy of Fallot) and neurosurgeon Dr. Walter Dandy, who pioneered the trigeminal rhizotomy.

Recognized as a leader in surgical oncology, Doris was one of 31 senior faculty members from schools of nursing across the country to be invited to a three-week Institute on Cancer Nursing. Rosalie Peterson, nurse officer of the Cancer Control Division of the National Institutes of Health, organized the program, which was held at the University of Minnesota in Minneapolis. Leading educators heard lectures, made clinical rounds, participated in discussion groups, and brain-stormed about ways to improve the nursing care available to patients with cancer. This course proved pivotal in identifying nursing leaders interested in promoting the practice of cancer nursing and in providing the impetus for future activities and grants.

The combination of nursing experience and exposure to the work of surgeons gave Doris an excellent background to help to write a textbook on surgical nursing. When Dr. Edward Stafford returned from Europe at the end of the war, he asked Doris to work with him on such a textbook. He had thought through the contents and recruited some of his military colleagues to help with the medical writing. Doris had been a nursing school classmate of Dr. Stafford's wife and a long-time family friend. An enduring physician-nurse writing team began with the first edition of *Textbook of Surgery for Nurses*, which was published by W.B. Saunders in 1947. In its foreword, Anna D. Wolf wrote,

Nursing as one branch of health services to the public, whether given in the home or hospital, has as a primary and fundamental concept that man is a social being; that all aspects of man's care in case of illness or in the maintenance of health bear upon the health and welfare of his family and community and must be directed toward his assumption of his social responsibilities. His illness and well-being reflect upon the national health. The professional nurse must assume her place as one of the team of co-operative experts in fulfilling this broad aspect of health service, irrespective of her particular locale or immediate activity. (p. iii)

The first edition was well received and adopted as the surgical nursing text in many schools of nursing. Two successive editions were published in 1954 and 1958. Each edition updated information about surgical procedures and the nurse's role in surgical care. Information about surgical recovery rooms was added to the second edition. A floor diagram that was included gave details down to lighting fixture wattage and locations of heavy-duty electrical outlets. The third edition contained a large section on radiation therapy. Each edition included excellent anatomic diagrams, procedural figures, and photographs. A typical drawing from the first edition is shown in Figure 1.

The following review of the third edition was published in *The Canadian Nurse.*

Surgery and Surgical Nursing by Edward S. Stafford, B.A., M.D., F.A.C.S. and Doris Diller, B.A., M.A., R.N., 469 pages. W.B. Saunders Company, East Washington Square, Philadelphia, PA, 3rd edition, 1958.

This is one of the outstanding surgical texts for nurses. The present revision has taken into account the general trend towards integration of subject material in the school of nursing curriculum.

General principles of surgery and surgical nursing care are discussed in the opening chapters. The succeeding chapters are devoted to specific anatomical areas in relation to the surgical conditions encountered and the care given. Two branches of surgery that are currently gaining significance in our general hospitals are discussed quite fully—cardiovascular and plastic surgery. In discussing surgery on the heart, the authors have also included the diagnostic procedures of the cardiac catheterization and cardioangiography.

The inclusion of a recovery room unit as part of the operating room suite is becoming an accepted feature of hospital facilities. Part of the chapter is devoted to a suggested plan for such a unit and the nursing care to be given in it. The special needs of the aged person who has had surgery and of the person with neoplastic disease received particular consideration.

This is an attractive and useful text. It is illustrated generously; headings and sub-headings provide easy identification of subject material; reference reading lists at the end of each chapter are adequate and up to date. This has been a very satisfactory student text in past years and should prove even more satisfactory in its present form. It is further recommended for the ward library and for the school of nursing library as a valuable reference text for nurses.

Note. From "Book Review of Surgery and Surgical Nursing," 1958, *The Canadian Nurse, 54,* p. 1144. Copyright 1958 by *The Canadian Nurse.* Reprinted with permission.

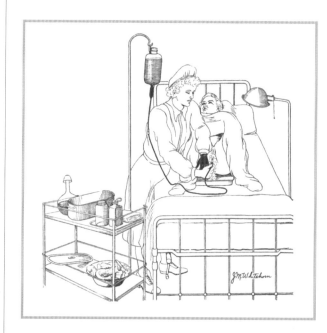

ABOVE
Figure 1. Irrigating the Perineal Wound Following Abdominoperineal Resection of the Rectum

Note. From *Textbook of Surgery for Nurses* (p. 274), by E.S. Stafford and D. Diller, 1947, Philadelphia: W.B. Saunders. Copyright 1947 by W.B. Saunders. Reprinted with permission.

DORIS DILLER

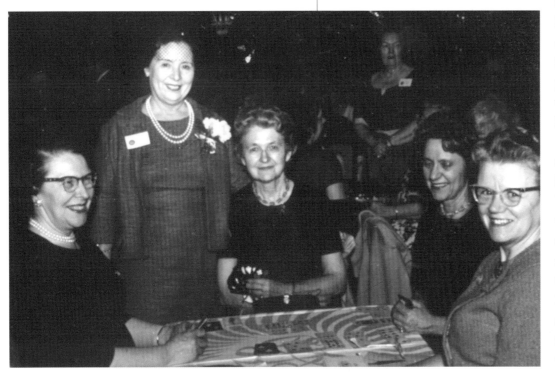

SKIDMORE COLLEGE

In August of 1952, Doris received a telegram from Skidmore College. The college had been awarded a grant from the National Cancer Institute (NCI) to integrate a cancer curriculum throughout the baccalaureate nursing program, and they were interested in talking to Doris about leading the work. She found the idea very appealing for several reasons. Doris had tremendous clinical experience and felt ready to share it with others outside The Johns Hopkins Hospital and its school. Doris also thought New York City would be a great place to live, having enjoyed the benefits of city living in Baltimore for several years. But probably the most compelling reason to consider Skidmore's offer was that no one had previously tried to do this work. For Doris, the excitement was in setting new directions. The grant was the first one for nursing education and was intended to address needs identified during the 1950s. Soon afterward, similar grants were awarded to Boston University, the University of California at Los Angeles, and Vanderbilt University. Washington University at St. Louis also was awarded a grant but withdrew from the program in 1955.

Doris moved to New York City in September of 1952 to begin work at Skidmore. She "didn't know a soul" but began to make friends through faculty members at school, and she took advantage of the city's activities. "It was wonderful," said Doris. After living temporarily in dormitory housing, she moved into an apartment at Peter Cooper Village and then into Stuyvesant Town, controlled housing for middle-income people. From this convenient location, she could walk to work and the clinical setting for the Skidmore students at New York University Medical Center.

Early in her time at Skidmore, Doris became concerned about being a faculty member without an advanced degree. She began working toward a master's degree at Columbia University and pondered over what research problem she would pursue. When implementing the Skidmore cancer curriculum grant, Doris asked herself and others about what nurses knew and what they ought to know. The idea of testing the cancer knowledge base took shape over time in Doris' mind and became her master's project, work that allowed her to apply for and receive research funding through NCI grants. She pursued test development courses with highly respected researchers in the areas of test development and measurement. She developed her testing approach and conducted pilot studies on students at various New York City nursing schools. Every three months she went to Washington to give progress reports on the Skidmore grant. She explained her testing project to one NCI official who told her, "You have a tiger by the tail. You have to expand this testing across the United States. This will raise the educational plane of nurses."

The testing program took hold and was funded on two additional submissions. At one point, Doris was testing 91 schools of nursing, both diploma and baccalaureate. Doris traveled to more than half the sites to administer the testing. She tried to live on the $13 per day that was the government per diem at the time and proudly noted that she was able to do so, except in Chicago. A common philosophy of the time was that students in diploma programs actually knew more than students in baccalaureate programs because diploma programs included far more direct patient care. The Diller study was expected to bear out this finding, but it did not. Another interesting aspect of the test was that one question continued to cause problems. Despite reworking of the question, the majority of students failed to correctly identify the reason that decompression of a distended bladder is performed gradually. Most students knew that gradual decompression was advisable, and many knew the upper limit of urine recommended for removal, but obtaining the correct answer, the why, evidently was not taught.

After completion of these major studies, Doris devoted her energies to teaching medical and surgical nursing to the Skidmore students. She became interested in the intensive care setting as it evolved and enjoyed introducing students to this level of care. She undertook some small research studies but did not publish the results. Her knowledge of surgical nursing and the visibility she achieved from her books and school study led to several speaking engagements, one of which was to provide a full week of neurology content to nurses in a hospital that was about to open a neurology service. Six years before her retirement, Doris was made a full-time professor—a real feat for a nurse without a doctoral degree.

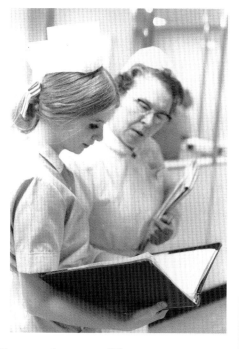

LEFT
Doris Diller
with nursing student
Candace Gerry
1971/72

Photo courtesy of Special Collections,
Lucy Scribner Library, Skidmore
College

BELOW
Doris Diller and a nursing
student

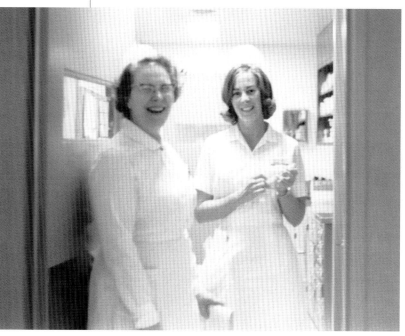

RETIREMENT

Doris retired at the age of 64, a year earlier than anticipated. She saw that the final year was going to put her back into an administrative role, and she knew from her earlier experience at Hopkins that she would hate it. She left New York City after her retirement and returned to Baltimore, where she had maintained a wide circle of friends. She was very active in work at her church, primarily in programs dealing with sheltering, clothing, and feeding the hungry and homeless. In 1972, she traveled to Europe, and in 1973, she toured the U.S. National Parks with a friend.

In 1989, Doris moved back to her native state of Ohio to be closer to family. "My brother said that when you are 80, it is time to head over the mountain and be near the relatives," she said. Having lived all of her adult life in a city, she was convinced that small-town living would not be to her liking. She settled in Columbus, OH, at the Westmont Thurber Center, a Presbyterian retirement center. She continues to be active in church work and raves about the services available in her community. In teacher fashion, she highlights key factors in selecting a retirement location. "Oh, you have to know what to look for in a retirement setting. The mobile post office, the bank representative, the library van, and the bus to go shopping are all important."

Currently, Doris' sewing machine is set up, and she is making a crazy quilt out of satins and velvets and darning a keepsake Quaker lace cloth for her church. She is an avid reader and boasts about her good eyesight and hearing. Her brother died in 1995, but his two daughters, their children, and their grandchildren visit her regularly. Four-year old triplets add to the merriment.

SUMMARY

The contributions of Doris Diller add an interesting dimension to understanding nursing and the emergence of cancer nursing. She went from a horse-and-cart town in rural Ohio to the heart of New York City. She went to college when most women of her age and station did not. She entered nursing school as a college graduate. She began her practice in the specialty of ophthalmology at a time when most new graduates were working as private-duty home nurses. She worked under two nursing giants, Elsie Lawler and Anna Wolf. She became a renowned clinical instructor, despite a lack of teaching instruction. She experienced and responded to the influences on health care of two major national events, the Depression and World War II. She developed procedures in surgical nursing to complement new surgical advances. For example, as Dr. Dandy developed new neurosurgical procedures, Doris wrote up care procedures by hand and left them in the recovery room to guide the patient care of the house staff and nurses. She never published these case notes, but they prepared her for writing the surgical textbooks. She traveled in a circle of New York City nurse leaders at a very exciting time, when specialization and advanced degrees were emerging. Her early admonishment to students to "always ask why" served her well throughout her profession and left a valuable legacy.

REFERENCES

Baird, S.B. (1987). A legacy unfolds. *ONS News, 2*(5), 1–2.

Craytor, J.K. (1985). Highlights in education for cancer nursing. In S.B. Baird & J.K. Brown (Eds.), *Oncology nursing recollections* (pp. 19–27). (Supplement to *Oncology Nursing Forum. 12*[1].)

Diller, Doris, interview by Susan Baird, 1987.

SELECTED WRITINGS
TEXTBOOK OF SURGERY FOR NURSES, 1ST EDITION (1947)
Chapter 4. Neoplastic Disease

A neoplasm is an adventitious growth of new tissue. Once thought to be parasitic upon the human body, neoplasms are now known to be composed of tissue cells originating from those of the person affected. Neoplastic disease seems to be the result of a local disturbance of the natural, orderly growth of cells, as though the usual regulating influences were not functioning properly. Thus the cells of a single region grow more rapidly and divide more frequently than normal, producing a local increase in tissue, or swelling, to which the ancients gave the name *tumor*.

Why tumors form is a subject not yet fully understood. Many theories have been advanced but none of them fits every case, nor is it likely that there is only one cause. One theory, which seems to explain the origin of many tumors, holds that the new tissue growth arises as the result of repeated interference with the natural process of repair. The growth of tumors in chronic ulcers and the production of tumors by chronic irritation, particularly by certain coal tar derivatives, are put forward in support of this theory. A second theory is that many tumors arise from small deposits of cells remaining from some developmental stage of the fetus, the embryonic rests. This theory affords a plausible explanation of such tumors as arise from the ovary and testis, and certain cystic tumors which will be discussed later; but no adequate reason is offered to explain why such cells produce a tumor occasionally but not always.

That neoplasms are due to an infectious agent has been suggested, and indeed there is in animals a tumor which is transmissible by a filtrable virus, the Rous chicken sarcoma. No evidence has been discovered, however, to show that any human tumor is transmissible or is due to any known infection.

Whether neoplastic disease is hereditary or not is a subject of controversy. It is certain that strains of mice may be bred which are less apt to develop spontaneous tumors than other strains. Human genetics cannot be reduced to simple terms, however, and where good records are obtainable there is seen to be scarcely any family without instances of neoplastic disease. The occurrence of similar tumors in many members of one family is not uncommon: yet such happenings may be coincidental and of no real significance from the standpoint of heredity.

Malignant Tumors

The very nature of malignant tumors constitutes a formidable obstacle to successful treatment. Just as in the case of benign tumors, the cure of a malignant neoplasm depends upon removal or destruction of the entire tumor. The extent of such tumors is not clearly defined, however, since there is malignant infiltration in every direction, and the surgeon may find it difficult to know how much tissue to remove. The occurrence of metastases, moreover, with the resultant growth of remotely situated daughter tumors, obviously precludes all possibility of cure. Added to these difficulties is another dread feature of malignancy, the insidious, symptomless onset of the tumor growth. Pain or other symptoms do not occur until the tumor has been present for a considerable time, and the unfortunate patient may be beyond all hope of cure before he feels the need of consulting a physician.

It is to be hoped that the time will come when the medical profession will have in its hands a method by which cancer in all stages can be cured. At present, however, the cure of malignant neoplastic disease depends upon early diagnosis, before metastasis has occurred, so that complete surgical removal or destruction by radiation may be accomplished.

Note. From "Neoplastic Diseases" (pp. 31–37) by D. Diller in E.S. Stafford and D. Diller (Eds.), *Textbook of Surgery for Nurses*, 1947, Philadelphia: W.B. Saunders Company. Copyright 1947 by W.B. Saunders Company. Excerpted with permission.

AN INVESTIGATION OF CANCER LEARNING IN NINETY-ONE SELECTED SCHOOLS OF NURSING (1957)

Knowledge of cancer as it applies to nursing has a wide scope including its nature, prevention, detection, diagnosis, treatment, nursing care and rehabilitation. In addition to the technical aspects, its bases are the biological sciences, physical sciences, social sciences and the humanities.[4] Cancer is one of the correlated major subjects in nursing and lends itself well to testing in many areas where the student nurse has opportunity to practice and learn.

The objective type of test was chosen at the most practical means to obtain information about the students' knowledge. There were other ways in which students' knowledge could have been obtained, such as interviews and observations, but these would have provided data on a more limited area of cancer knowledge; also, objectivity would have been influenced by the opinions of the persons giving the test.[2]

The development of the test to measure cancer knowledge on the part of nurses involved two kinds of problems. Identifying the information was difficult because cancer knowledge as it applies to nursing is not available in textbook form in contrast to much of the content in nursing educa-

DORIS DILLER

tion. Therefore, this information had to be obtained from various sources including books, periodicals and the judgment of many people. The construction of the text itself was another problem which necessitated the development of relevant items and options which would separate good from poor students. There have been gradual changes in the test items and options to increase the validity of the test.

The National Cancer Institute made a grant to Skidmore College to provide for testing students in approximately one hundred schools of nursing whose distribution covered a wide geographic area in the United States. The aim was to help nurse educators evaluate this area of learning in their schools. It was anticipated at the time the grant was made that this study would be carried out during 1955, 1956, and 1957.

The multiplicity of educational programs in schools of nursing throughout the nation is acknowledged and therefore, the strict systematic comparison of all levels of students from school to school, except the senior students, is difficult. The data obtained for each school at all levels tested can be interpreted by the individual school, through correlation of learning activities of the students and their test results, to evaluate the attainment of their students at this particular level. The senior or third year scores furnish data for comparing one school with another in their respective kind of educational level.

The essential purposes of this study were therefore:

1. To develop a valid and reliable cancer knowledge test for nurses.
2. To measure as accurately as possible the breadth and depth of cancer knowledge as it applies to nursing.
3. To measure growth of knowledge for each school at different levels of education.

Summary, Conclusions and Hypotheses

A written multiple choice type test on the subject of cancer, as it applies to nursing, was developed. In 1955, 1956 and 1957 a total of over twenty-five thousand student nurses enrolled in diploma and basic degree programs took this test. A report of the average scores of student groups in their respective levels of education in the program was sent to each school which participated. Charts revealing the averages of all schools were sent to provide comparative data. The scores of each student were also sent to each school. In addition, the first, second and final reports of the investigation were also sent to each school. Each year, the individual scores of faculty members who took the test were sent to all who indicated their name and address.

The validity and reliability of the test were satisfactory for measuring cancer knowledge as it applies to nursing, according to a number of criteria. The validity has increased during the three years, according to the criteria listed. The statistics showed that groups of students were more homogeneous after the first investigation in 1955.

Some of the conclusions which were reached through the investigation of the results follow.

Each year, the most significant gain in cancer knowledge occurred during the second year in diploma and basic degree programs. There were several general impressions gained during this investigation of the responses to questions by students and faculty.

Students in both programs have repeatedly scored high on questions dealing with the early symptoms of cancer publicized by the American Cancer Society. However, when these were related to the discovery of early cancer in different body sites where detection can be made through an ordinary physical examination (including a vaginal and rectal examination without use of any instruments) the scores were significantly lower for all students. The relationship of early detection of common types of cancer to physical examination would be a good area for further study. The gain in information concerning cancer as it applies to nursing from the first to third year in diploma schools revealed that it was greatest for the categories of nervous system, endocrine system, and leukemia and lymphoma in 1956 and 1957.

The gain in information from the freshman to senior year in the basic degree programs was greatest each year in the nervous system.

In 1955, 1956, and 1957 the questions relating to the male genital system were the most difficult for both diploma and basic degree students. In 1957, both the diploma and basic degree students showed a larger gain than in the two preceding years. Knowledge of cancer of the male genital tract evidently presents the most difficulty and also showed the poorest gain of all the anatomical sites. Several of the questions related to the action of drugs; students found these difficult. This led to the examination of all questions relating to action of drugs. It was found that these were more difficult items than any groups of questions examined. The cause of the confusion or poor knowledge concerning the action of drugs would be a good field for investigation.

Even though a test meets the criteria of validity and reliability, the number of questions is limited, and therefore, data pertaining to specific categories of cancer learning should be considered only as pointers of weaknesses or strengths. Such pointers can be followed up by the faculty to obtain more adequate information regarding the knowledge in specific categories.

References

1. Adkins, Dorothy C. *Construction and Analysis of Achievement Tests*. Washington, D.C.: U.S. Printing Office, U.S. Civil Service Commission, 1947.

2. Bierman, Howard and others. *Cancer Learning in the Medical School*. Berkeley, California: The University of California Press, 1953.

3. Diller, Doris. *An Investigation of Cancer Learning in Ninety-One Selected Schools of Nursing*. Second Report. New York. Skidmore College, Department of Nursing, 1957.

4. Leone, Lucille Petry. "The Art of Nursing." *J.A.M.A.*, 157:1381–1383 (April 16, 1955).

5. Lindquist, E.F. (Editor). *Educational Measurement*. Washington, D.C.: American Council on Education, 1951.

6. National Cancer Institute. *Cancer Nursing in the Basic Professional Nursing Curriculum*. Washington Printing Office, 1951.

7. Richardson, M.W., and Kuder, G.F. "The Calculation of Test Reliability Coefficient Based on the Method of Rationale Equivalence." *J. Ed. Psych.*, 30:681–687 (1939).

8. *Statistics on Cancer, New York City*. New York: American Cancer Society, 1952.

Note. From *An Investigation of Cancer Learning in Ninety-One Selected Schools of Nursing* (pp. 1–26) , by D. Diller, 1957, New York: Skidmore College Department of Nursing. Copyright 1957 by Skidmore College Department of Nursing. Excerpted with permission.

A CANCER KNOWLEDGE TEST FOR NURSES (1958)

Where does cancer rank among the leading causes of death in the United States?

a. Fourth.

b. Third.

c. Second.

d. First.

Metastases usually do <u>not</u> occur by means of

a. lymphatic system.

b. portal system.

c. arterial circulation.

d. nervous system.

Which of the following substances in industry is <u>not</u> known to incite cancer?

a. Soot.

b. Petroleum.

c. Arsenicals.

d. Silver.

To aid case-finding and early diagnosis of childhood cancer, which of the following would be most likely to have significance?

a. Drooping of one eye lid.

b. Solid mass.

c. Abdominal pain.

d. Vomiting after food consumption.

A treatment which is not considered useful in the cure of any cancer is

a. radioactive iodine.

b. X-ray.

c. cobra venom.

d. cobalt bomb.

The earliest sign or symptom of cancer of the esophagus usually is

a. hematemesis.

b. dysphagia.

c. persistent chronic indigestion.

d. regurgitation.

Surgeons are in general agreement that a radical mastectomy for breast cancer is not the treatment of choice when

a. the tumor has been present for ten months or longer.

b. the axillary nodes on the side of the tumor can be palpated.

c. there has been a bloody discharge from the nipple prior to biopsy.

d. an extension of the tumor is present in the lung.

The first sign of Hodgkin's disease is usually

a. swelling of the cervical nodes.

b. loss of weight and fatigue.

c. recurrent attacks of fever.

d. high eosinophil count.

Which of the following reactions most frequently occurs while the patient is taking sulfasuxidine or sulfathalidine?

a. Nausea and vomiting.

b. Erythema.

c. Diarrhea.

d. Excessive dryness of the mouth.

One desired effect of the administration of estrogens in patients with advanced carcinoma of the prostate is to

a. relieve pain.

b. prevent urethral strictures.

c. increase the functioning of the prostate gland.

d. lessen the action of thyroid gland.

Note. From *A Cancer Knowledge Test for Nurses* (pp. 1–16), by D. Diller, 1958, New York: Skidmore College Department of Nursing. Copyright 1958 by Skidmore College Department of Nursing. Excerpted with permission.

TRIBUTE

Although many years have passed since I have seen Doris Diller, when you ask me about her, I hold this vivid image of when we were both teaching at The Johns Hopkins Hospital.

I was one of the few faculty members at The Johns Hopkins School of Nursing who had not graduated from the school. When I arrived in the early 1940s, I knew no one, was not familiar with the layout of the hospital, and certainly did not have any idea about the policies, personalities, or the politics. I remember how kind Doris was in helping me through the maze and making me feel welcome. She was someone I could count on, and I knew that I could go to her with my questions.

I taught Fundamentals of Nursing to the incoming student nurses, after which they went on to learn Surgical Nursing from Doris. She had the reputation of being an excellent teacher and was well respected by the surgical staff at the hospital. She was slow and deliberate in the manner in which she expressed herself. This caused you to listen and think about her views. She had many good ideas and always was optimistic about solving problems.

Doris was one of those faculty members whom you could count on, both personally and professionally. Even back in the 1940s, she was a leader among the staff at Johns Hopkins.

Eleanor Hall, RN, MA

Former Dean and Professor Emeritus
University of Rochester
School of Nursing
Rochester, NY

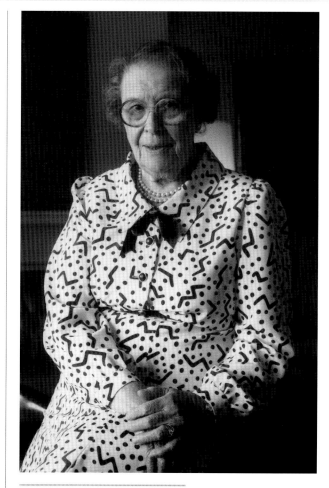

ABOVE
Doris Diller

VIRGINIA BARCKLEY, RN, MS
Leader in Advocating for Cancer Nursing Through Education and Scholarships

"Those were the days when you did more than you had to do . . . because you knew that working for what you believed in surpassed any other satisfaction in the world."

—*Virginia Barckley*

VIRGINIA BARCKLEY

SIGNIFICANT CAREER CONTRIBUTIONS

- Wrote *The Play's the Thing,* a collection of skits and discussions in nursing, which was published by the League of Nursing in 1959
- Created a program to improve the care of patients with cancer in nursing homes
- Designed a milestone project with the Instructive Visiting Nurse Association of Richmond, VA, in which a visiting nurse identified as a cancer specialist gave patients care at home
- Developed a work-study program in cancer nursing to expand the clinical experience of student nurses
- Laid the groundwork for a curriculum guide for a master's degree in cancer nursing and nursing scholarships
- Authored *Cancer Nursing: Information and Concepts,* a manual that has been widely used by nurses in developing countries

LEFT
Virginia Barckley and father
George Force Barckley

RIGHT
Barckley children
Virginia and brother James
Wilson

BIOGRAPHICAL INFORMATION
BIRTH AND DEATH

Virginia Barckley was born on November 19, 1911, in Burlington, NJ. She died January 15, 1993, at her apartment in New York City, at the age of 82.

PARENTS

Virginia's father was George Force Barckley, who worked as a foundry inspector in a pipe-making plant in Burlington. Her mother, Ethel Smith, was born in New Jersey. Ethel was a homemaker who was skilled at painting, decorating, and upholstery and was involved in local church activities. George and Ethel met and married in New Jersey and resided in Burlington.

FAMILY

Virginia was born second of two children. Her older brother, James Wilson, became a biochemist. He married and had two daughters. When his wife died at an early age, he and his two daughters, ages 14 and 12, moved back to live with his parents. George and Ethel raised the two girls. Virginia chose nursing as a career and left home for nurse's training at age 18. She never married.

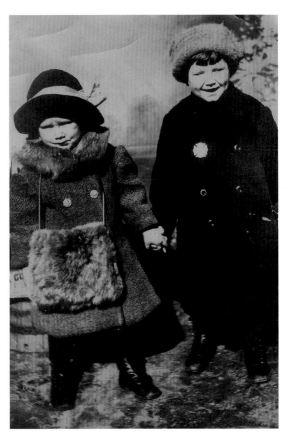

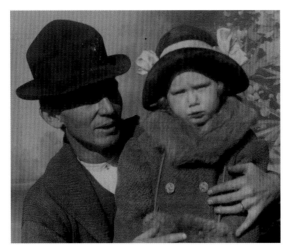

CAREER PATH

Virginia completed her nurse's training in the early 1940s at Flushing Hospital in New York. She earned a bachelor's degree in nursing from the University of Pennsylvania in 1943. While attending school, Virginia gained experience as a homecare nurse by working on the staff of the Philadelphia Visiting Nurse Association. Between 1943 and 1957, she worked in a variety of positions, including staff nurse, head nurse, supervising nurse, public health coordinator, and mental health nurse for agencies and institutions located in New Jersey, Michigan, New York, and Pennsylvania. By combining work and school, Virginia received a master's degree in mental health nursing from Catholic University in Washington, DC.

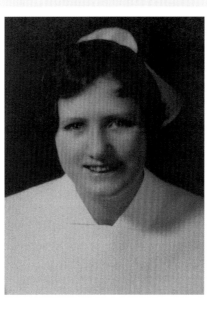

LEFT
Virginia Barckley as a student nurse

BELOW
Virginia Barckley during her work as a visiting nurse

PENNSYLVANIA STATE DEPARTMENT OF HEALTH

In 1957, the Pennsylvania State Department of Health appointed Virginia as its Mental Health Nursing Consultant, a position that she held until 1962. Shortly after becoming a nurse, she chose to become a volunteer for the American Cancer Society (ACS). In spite of her many moves and job changes, Virginia continued to contribute her time and service as a dedicated volunteer.

AMERICAN CANCER SOCIETY

In 1962, ACS offered Virginia the position of National Nurse Consultant. This position, which had been established in 1944, was the avenue for coordinating nursing activities within ACS. During the next 14 years, Virginia gave tirelessly of her time and expertise to promoting cancer nursing.

Diseases are as individual as the patients who have them, but cancer especially seems to have a set of fingerprints all its own. To many patients, cancer means extreme pain, to some, disfigurement or change in body function, and to almost all, a serious threat to survival. Few other illnesses combine so tragically the wearing qualities of a long illness with the tearing qualities of an acute one. (Barckley, 1967, p. 278)

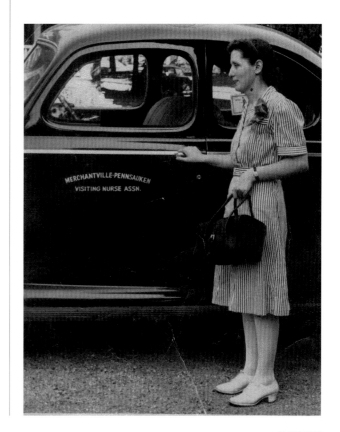

VIRGINIA BARCKLEY

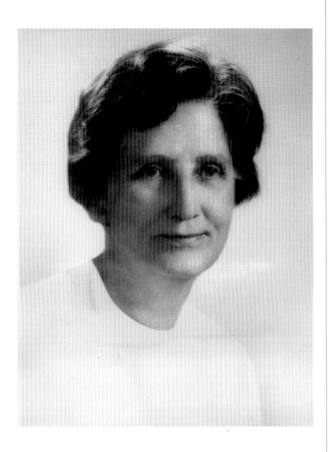

ABOVE
Virginia Barckley
National Nurse Consultant
American Cancer Society

Virginia traveled to all 50 states and many foreign countries in her capacity as professional educator and service provider for ACS. In collaboration with members of the ACS Nursing Advisory Committee, she implemented a number of innovative programs for improving nurses' skills and knowledge of cancer. ACS's work-study program, which she and Renilda Hilkemeyer, nursing director at M.D. Anderson Cancer Center in Texas, initiated in cooperation with Memorial Sloan-Kettering Cancer Center and M.D. Anderson Cancer Center, was the first of these innovations. This program gave student nurses clinical experience in cancer nursing through internships at various cancer centers.

As a cancer nurse consultant, she provided guidance, in-service education, individual problem-solving sessions, and encouragement to nursing home personnel in the Miami area. In 1963, Virginia pioneered another nursing innovation for improving cancer care. In collaboration with the Dade County unit of the Florida division of ACS, the Nursing Home Cancer Care Improvement Program was launched. The following quote is taken from notes Virginia used in preparing a speech on cancer in the aged. It highlights her concern for the older person with cancer.

Cancer is a disease of older people. No illness and no host is more provocative, or more appealing to nursing's compassion, energy, resources, and response to challenges. Nurses who work with older patients have always found there is more to their commitment than giving. They receive glimpses of dignity, valor, and wisdom that only a long span of years can bring, a luminous gift.
(Barckley, from speech notes on cancer in the aged)

Because of her public health background, Virginia was aware of the many needs of homebound patients with cancer. This insight led her to initiate another ACS-funded project, which she carried out under the direction of the Instructive Visiting Nurses Association of Richmond, VA. The expertise of a cancer nurse specialist was used to help consult nurses caring for homebound patients with cancer. These two programs, in nursing homes and in the home, were among the earliest endeavors that created a unique role for a cancer nurse specialist.

Nursing school faculty members were another nursing group that Virginia targeted, recognizing that they needed the latest information about cancer. Her innovative response to this need was to create an ACS scholarship program that provided nursing faculty with the opportunity to attend a continuing-education course. Classes were held at cancer centers during the summer months, when faculty members were free from their teaching responsibilities.

In 1973, another significant educational endeavor was set in motion. Virginia, along with Renilda, organized the first National Conference on Cancer Nursing. They had expected a maximum of 100 nurses to attend and were amazed when they learned that 2,500 nurses had registered. This conference was one of the catalysts that led to the establishment of the Oncology Nursing Society (ONS).

In 1979, Virginia led the group of educators in laying the foundation of a curriculum guide for obtaining a specialty in cancer nursing at the master's level. Later, ACS established its nursing scholarship program, which has funded education for hundreds of nurses at the master's and doctoral levels since 1981.

Recognition of Virginia's leadership in cancer nursing extended into the international community. The World Health Organization invited Virginia and Renilda to organize the first cancer nursing conference in Peru. Based on requests from the Peruvian nurses, a very practical clinically based program was planned. Again, the number of nurses who attended the conference exceeded their expectations. In 1978, Virginia chaired the first nursing workshop held in conjunction with the International Union Against Cancer (UICC) in Argentina. The worldwide need for cancer information was apparent, and, with Virginia's encouragement, ACS responded. She authored the manual *Cancer Nursing: Information and Concepts*, and UICC distributed it to cancer nurses in developing countries.

Throughout her lifetime, Virginia was a prolific writer, contributing to professional journals, ACS publications, and textbooks. She was a sought-after speaker who was skilled at delivering her message by painting vivid pictures through storytelling. Motivating young oncology nurses was one of her unique talents. Nurses from around the country can testify to receiving handwritten notes of encouragement. Others recall words of support that she offered to them personally.

BELOW
Virginia Barckley (center)
XIIth International Cancer Congress
Buenos Aires, Argentina
1978

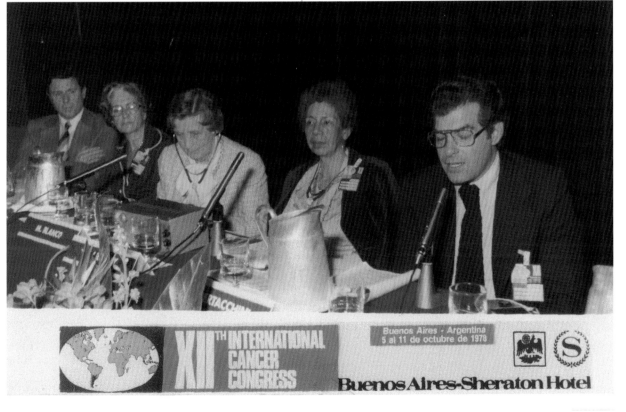

VIRGINIA BARCKLEY

Some doctors reveal the diagnosis of cancer; some hide it from almost all patients; some act on a strictly individual basis. Whatever the doctor's decision, the nurse supports it, so that the patient will not be caught between opposing philosophies.

BARCKLEY, 1967, P. 279

Virginia received numerous awards and citations, starting with the 1961 Citation Merit presented to her by the Pennsylvania division of ACS for "service to the cause of cancer control." In 1981, Virginia became an honorary member of the Association of Pediatric Oncology Nurses. ONS put forth the following resolution that acknowledged her contributions to cancer nursing:

Oncology Nursing Society
Resolution #4
Title: A Commemorative Resolution to Acknowledge
the Leadership of Virginia Barckley, RN, MS, in Oncology Nursing

Whereas: Oncology nursing has emerged as a recognized specialty of professional nursing; and

Whereas: There are recognized nurse leaders who have contributed to the advancement of this specialty in education, practice, and research; and

Whereas: These nurses have recognized the unique nursing care needs of cancer patients and families and developed appropriate nursing care criteria; and

Whereas: These nurses recognized the unique nursing education needs of both nurses entering the profession and those within the profession; and

Whereas: Nurses practicing in this specialty acknowledge the pioneering efforts of these nursing leaders; therefore, be it

Resolved: *That the Oncology Nursing Society acknowledge one of these leaders, Virginia Barckley, RN, MS, for her foresight, leadership, and contributions to the development of oncology nursing education and practice.*

Sponsored by	Education Committee
Endorsed by	Judith L. Johnson, RN, PhD
	Barbara Piper, RN, MS
	Jean Brown, RN, MS
	Rachel E. Spector, RN, MS

May 1981

In 1984, Memorial Sloan-Kettering Cancer Center awarded Virginia its Centennial Medal for Lifelong Achievement. At the presentation, Dr. Paul Marks said, "Your character and gentleness, your dedication and devotion have been inspirational to generations of nurses and has endeared you to your colleagues the world over." In 1986, the International Society of Nurses in Cancer Care gave their prestigious Distinguished Merit Award to Virginia in recognition of her many contributions to cancer nursing worldwide.

After retiring in 1986, Virginia returned home to her apartment in New York City. She took an interest in tutoring young children in a local grammar school. She also enjoyed decorating the lobby of her apartment complex during holidays, especially for the Christmas season. Unfortunately, a number of chronic health problems gradually compromised her health and set limits on her activities. These problems led to a hospitalization for pneumonia, which left Virginia frail and requiring assistance. Thanks to the help of her niece, Ann Callahan, she was able to return home. After five months of care, Virginia died on January 15, 1993, at the age of 82.

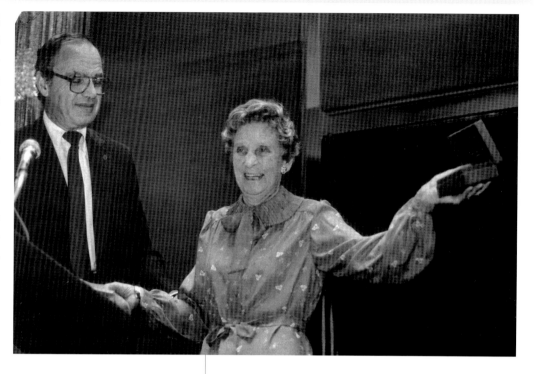

ABOVE
Dr. Paul Marks presenting Virginia with the Memorial Sloan-Kettering Cancer Center's Centennial Medal for Lifelong Achievement
1984

SUMMARY

Virginia, who became a volunteer for ACS in the 1940s and later served as their National Nurse Consultant, dedicated more than 40 years of her professional career to ACS and the specialty of cancer nursing. She was one of a handful of nurses throughout the country who believed in the contributions nursing could make to the care of patients with cancer. She wanted to expand nurses' knowledge and share their expertise. This belief led her to initiate national conferences on cancer nursing and promoting education and scholarships for nurses on the undergraduate and graduate levels. Virginia's commitment to improving care for people with cancer resulted in the development of innovative programs that used cancer nurse specialists in the homecare setting and in nursing homes. Her poignant writings and storytelling approach to delivering speeches were her trademark. She undoubtedly has touched the lives of generations of cancer nurses throughout the world.

VIRGINIA BARCKLEY

If we are sure of our own feelings, if we have some central core of philosophy to rely on, then this is reflected in our manner with patients. The precise phrases we use, when we have emphathy, are not important. We need not learn a speech, for the words will come.

BARCKLEY, 1958, P. 316

REFERENCES

Barckley, V. (1958). What can I say to the cancer patient? *Nursing Outlook, 6*(6), 316.

Barckley, V. (1967). The crisis in cancer. *American Journal of Nursing, 67*, 278–280.

Barckley, V. (1970). A visiting nurse specializes in cancer nursing. *American Journal of Nursing, 70*, 1680–1683.

Barckley, V. (1970). Cancer consultant to nursing homes. *American Journal of Nursing, 70*, 804–806.

Barckley, V. (1985). The best of times and the worst of times: Historical reflections from an American Cancer Society national consultant. *Oncology Nursing Forum, 12*(Suppl. 1), 16–18.

Haylock, P. (2000). *American nursing: A biographical dictionary.* New York: Springer.

Marks, P. (1984). Virginia Barckley gets cancer award. *Public Health Highlights, 5*(12), 1.

Zanca, J. (1993). Virginia Barckley: A lifetime of service, as told by her lifelong friend, Renilda Hilkemeyer. *Cancer Nursing News, 4*(11), 1–2.

Callahan, Ann, interview by Judith Johnson, May 1999.

SELECTED WRITINGS

EXCERPTS FROM VIRGINIA BARCKLEY'S SPEECH
CANCER IN AN AGING SOCIETY

What can cancer nursing do? We can initiate a bold comprehensive nursing program of teaching care and support that begins with prevention and extends through death and bereavement visits, and includes student affiliations and evaluation. Somewhere in this plan will come a discovery of what the aged contribute to younger people; as role models and teachers they are incomparable. How do we do all this? By combining the specialties of gerontologic nursing with oncologic nursing, by including nutritionists, clergymen, physical therapists, social workers, dentists and volunteers to join in the effort.

The reasons for involving other disciplines are obvious. Public health nurses have always observed that most communities have more patient services available than are known or used. It is the coordination that is off stroke. We need the knowledge, ability, and feeling of dozens of experts to develop a tenable approach to a problem of the dimensions of cancer and aging. Yet it is important for nursing to escape the sharp delineation that sometimes relegates it to the dispensing of pills or the passing of nasogastric tubes. Because of our unique closeness to patients, and because nursing is still the discipline that is on duty nights, weekends, and holidays, it is to us that troubled patients turn most.

We can examine our own attitudes toward the aging—are they tinged with distaste and impatience? Do we see the enormous strengths of those in whom a process of natural selectivity has occurred? Many older people have the wisdom accrued from experience and the compassion that may develop from deep suffering. They bear pain well, they respond to touch and loving care in ways that show us how long they have been without the human concern so necessary to life beyond the most basic level.

Nurses who work with older patients have always found there is more to their commitment than giving. They receive glimpses of dignity, valor and wisdom that only a long span of years can bring, a luminous gift.

I urge all nurses here today to think more about their older cancer patients and to do more for them. If this isn't your problem now, it will be, for the whole cancer world is evolving. No path could be more rewarding.

Note. From *Cancer in an Aging Society* by V. Barckley. Excerpts from preparatory notes from personal file.

VIRGINIA BARCKLEY

THE CRISIS IN CANCER (1967)

Diseases are as individual as the patients who have them, but cancer, especially, seems to have a set of fingerprints all its own. To many patients, cancer means extreme pain; to some, disfigurement or a change in body function; and to almost all, a serious threat to survival. Cancer is also characterized by the specter of recurrence, no small one. The disease pervades every life area, so that even those who are not concerned by the heavy expenses incurred may be distraught over its effect on a loved family member, on a career, or on social acceptability. Few other illnesses combine so tragically the wearing qualities of a long illness with the tearing qualities of an acute one.

Most of all, cancer has a bad name. Some of us were brought up where the word was too dreadful to mention, so we resorted to euphemisms, referring to our neighbors' "growths" or "tumors." Their deaths were not ascribed to a particular cause, but were announced as "following a long illness." This stigma probably began with the premise that illness was punishment for evil; hence, the wrongdoing that produced cancer was obviously greater than the peccadilloes resulting in grippe.

All the suffering from cancer does not fall to the lot of the patient. Whether they are loving or incompatible, the well people in the family are involved, though for different reasons and to different degrees. The extraordinary limits of human endurance are often demonstrated by relatives who expend themselves on trips to hospital, doctor, and drugstore, on extra cooking, laundry, cleaning, and personal care, interlarded with fear, worry, and indebtedness—all on a heroic scale.

Whatever the crisis for the patient, loving relatives—and, sometimes, merely dutiful ones—share it. Obviously their need for support is tremendous. Much of it can and does come from nurses, who, in spite of a tendency to underrate themselves, have unusual opportunities and abilities to help troubled people.

Finally, it may be comforting to reflect on the word, "crisis," which has an ominous connotation for many of us. Decades ago, the crisis in pneumonia or typhoid fever was a dreaded peak that for some patients preceded death. But it also meant the turning point. Now, too, with caring, crisis can be the harbinger, not of despair, but of new strength and serenity.

Note. From "The Crisis in Cancer" by V. Barckley, 1967, *American Journal of Nursing, 67,* 278–280. Copyright 1967 by American Journal of Nursing Company. Excerpted with permission.

TRIBUTES

I first met Virginia Barckley in 1973 when I attended the first American Cancer Society (ACS) conference on cancer nursing in Chicago. At that time, I was president of APON, the Association of Pediatric Oncology Nurses, and had just finished graduate school at the University of Florida. I was working at Grady Hospital in Atlanta as a clinical nurse specialist in pediatric oncology. Of course, I was familiar with Virginia through her prolific writings in the *American Journal of Nursing*. Very little was written about cancer, and Virginia's work was the mainstay of cancer information for nurses at the bedside.

Out of that conference, the National Nursing Advisory Committee for ACS was formed. A previous committee existed in the 1950s, but a group of nurses wasn't committed to see it survive. In the 1970s, the times had changed, and the National Cancer Act had been signed into law. New interest was shown in establishing cancer as a specialty in medicine and nursing. Virginia had a vision to increase the resources for nurses to care for patients. She was the Nurse Consultant for ACS, and, in that role, she developed a number of special projects that the Advisory Committee reviewed and recommended. We met as a group several times a year to evaluate existing programs and review proposals for new ones. Virginia was committed to establishing nursing within ACS on equal footing with medicine. One of Virginia's greatest skills was that she was able to transmit information to the masses to meet their needs. Virginia opened the door for the range of programs that has been established over the years, the ACS professorships, master's-level scholarships, doctoral scholarships, and nursing research conferences. Virginia remains an inspiration to me. What I admired about her the most was her tireless energy and her outward focus on others. In 1981, when I was asked to replace Virginia as the Nurse Consultant at ACS, I knew that it would be a challenge to fill her shoes and preserve the spirit of her work. Our positions at ACS did not overlap, so I never had the opportunity to work directly with her. However, she taught me a great deal at our committee meetings, and the structure she left in place at ACS helped to advance us in ways that none of us realized at the time. Virginia helped others to realize the special skills that nurses bring to patients that other professionals cannot provide.

Trish Greene, RN, PhD, FAAN

Senior Vice President
Leukemia Society of America
New York, NY
(This tribute was the last thing penned by Trish Greene before her death from pancreatic cancer in August 1999.)

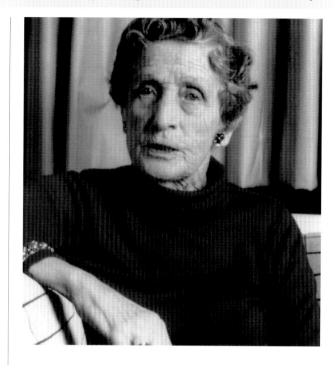

ABOVE
Virginia Barckley

VIRGINIA BARCKLEY

Although I never met Virginia Barckley, she has had a profound influence on my professional life. Virginia was instrumental in the creation and development of the National Institutes of Health (NIH) Nursing Internship Program and the American Cancer Society (ACS) Grant Program for Graduate Nursing Study.

After several careers, including teaching biology and selling pharmaceuticals, I returned to college to pursue a degree in nursing. By the beginning of my senior year, I was experiencing the frustration of the disconnection between what I was learning in school and how nursing was practiced. Once again, I was concerned that I had chosen the wrong career path. Then I applied for and was accepted by the NIH Nursing Internship Program. I chose to do my internship at the National Cancer Institute (NCI) where my preceptors, Jean Jenkins and Ricky Preston, role modeled nursing the way I was taught it should be. At NCI, I also was exposed to a "new" nursing organization, the Oncology Nursing Society. With renewed enthusiasm, I returned to college and completed my degree.

Following graduation, I started my nursing career on Masonic III, the leukemia unit at the University of Minnesota. I had found my career niche and it felt "right." Confident that I finally had found a career I loved, I wanted to pursue a master's degree in oncology nursing. Once again, the influence of Virginia opened a door for me—the ACS Grant Program for Graduate Nursing.

The study provided an $8,000 renewable grant to pursue a master's degree in oncology nursing. I was awarded one of the grants and attended the University of Rochester.

Now, in my 21st year of oncology nursing practice, having held many different positions in a variety of settings, there are many people who deserve special acknowledgment. Virginia Barckley is one of those people.

It is an honor to be able to recognize Virginia. The NIH Nursing Internship Program and the ACS Grant Program for Graduate Nursing Study are just two examples of the many ways she promoted the growth of oncology nursing and contributed to improved care of patients with cancer.

Cathy Berendts, RN, MS, AOCN®

Director
Saint Mary's Duluth Clinic
Cancer Center
Duluth, MN

Professional papers and effects of Virginia Barckley are located in the archives at the National Office of the Oncology Nursing Society in Pittsburgh, PA.

RENILDA E. HILKEMEYER, RN, BS, DPS
Leader in Administration and Clinical Practice in Cancer Nursing

"I do not believe it is good for us to live in the past, but I believe there is merit in looking at the past in order to have a perspective of accomplishments, challenges, trends, and future needs. Moreover, I think it can give us the courage and determination to pursue our ideas and ideals . . . I believe nurses who were involved in cancer nursing in the past can be proud of the heritage which they established in this field."

— Renilda E. Hilkemeyer

RENILDA E. HILKEMEYER

SIGNIFICANT CAREER CONTRIBUTIONS

- Pioneer in developing on-site continuing-education courses in cancer nursing at Ellis Fischel State Cancer Hospital in Missouri

- Served as the director of the Department of Nursing and promoted oncology nursing at the University of Texas M.D. Anderson Hospital and Tumor Institute in Houston

- Represented cancer nursing through key roles at the American Cancer Society, National Cancer Institute, and National Institutes of Health

- Received an honorary doctoral degree, Doctor of Public Service, in 1988 from St. Louis University, MO

- First recipient of the Distinguished Merit Award for National and International Contributions from the International Society of Nurses in Cancer Care

BIOGRAPHICAL INFORMATION

BIRTH

Renilda E. Hilkemeyer was born on July 29, 1915, in Martinsburg, MO.

PARENTS

Renilda was the second child of Henry Gerald and Anna Marie Bertels Hilkemeyer, hardworking people of German heritage. Henry ran a livery stable in town and also drove a trade wagon delivering packages and heavy shipments from the train station to area businesses. He rented surreys to young men so they could impress their dates and also to make sure they got home safely. "The horses always knew the way back," noted Renilda. When the livery business decreased with the influx of cars, Renilda's father and older brother Edmond went into the building industry. They built houses and often were away from home for long periods of time.

Renilda described her mother as a woman "ahead of her time." She was a homemaker and an excellent seamstress. She made all of the children's clothing and could copy any garment she saw. When Renilda's mother was over the age of 50, she heard about a dress factory where sewers were being hired. She got on the bus, got the job, and worked at the company for more than five years. Anna Marie always had a large vegetable garden and canned vegetables for the winter. Renilda remembered buying a freezer for her mother—a major purchase from the salary of her first nursing job—to make things easier for her. Anna Marie was a member of the County Democratic Committee and involved the children in distributing notices and campaign information around town. Renilda's mother often was described as "moving all the time," and Renilda's sister later said that Renilda was the same way.

FAMILY

Renilda and her two brothers and sister grew up in Martinsburg, MO, a rural Catholic town of approximately 7,000 people. The town was primarily made up of tradesmen, and the surrounding areas were given to farming, with people growing grain and raising horses. After church, a favorite Sunday activity for the children was to go to their grandparents' farm. They fought over who was going to get to go, and they hated to come back home. Renilda attended the local parochial grammar school and attended public school for the first two years of high school. For her final two years of school, Renilda attended a Roman Catholic high school, which was 17 miles away. She stayed with a local divorced woman, who worked for an ophthalmologist, and helped to take care of her children. Renilda found herself helping out in the ophthalmologist's office on Saturdays. The doctor asked Renilda what she thought she was going to do after high school and told her that she should consider nursing because he felt that she was very good with people.

Renilda's mother had siblings who were living in St. Louis, so Renilda traveled there and attended St. Mary's Hospital School of Nursing. Students in this program took some of their classes at St. Mary's but also took some courses such as anatomy and physiology at St. Louis University with the medical students. As was typical of this time, students were essential to the staffing of the hospital, especially on the off shifts. Renilda noted that St. Mary's was a good school but questioned, "How did we survive?" Students frequently were responsible for 36-bed wards on the off shifts, and their supervisors often were nuns, who were their fellow students. They lived in dormitories, with a housemother overseeing their comings and goings. They had one half day a week off from classes and floor duty. Renilda was known for being able to sleep easily at any time and could withstand juggling night duty and day classes, so she often was called on for night duty. Renilda attributed this experience as the basis for her organizational skills. "I had to learn to organize to get through the shift. We had to make sure everybody got turned, rolled, and pillowed. We had to do the sterilizing and pass the wash water." She took care of patients with cancer, but they were not referred to as "cancer patients." Instead, these patients stayed on the floor for patients who were terminally ill. They also were scattered among the surgery patients. Cancer was not an area of interest for Renilda at that time.

Renilda never married. "Not that I didn't have opportunities," she said, "but I looked at what I wanted to do and just never acted on those opportunities." As adults, her siblings scattered. Her older brother, Edmond Gerard, had very bad asthma and moved to Arizona for a more favorable climate. Her sister, Mary Jane, moved with her husband to Iowa. Her younger brother, Gerald Francis, stayed at home. He worked hauling cattle to market and later owned his own trucking company, the Hilkemeyer Trucking Company. He became sick and was diagnosed with a Pancoast tumor at M.D. Anderson Hospital. He took part in a research project, in which he received radiation therapy, and he did well for about three-and-a-half years.

Within a five-year period, Edmond died of complications from his asthma, and Renilda's mother and her brother Gerald also died. When her sister, Mary Jane, retired, she went back to Texas and currently lives near Renilda. Nieces and nephews are a very important part of Renilda's life. One niece works for Dr. Denton Cooley, the famous heart surgeon, and has been taking care of his papers and publications for more than 13 years. A nephew is the family historian and keeps track of all of Renilda's accomplishments. A great-niece is a student at Texas A&M University and plans to pursue a career in veterinary medicine.

When diagnosis has been established, the question arises as to what the cancer patient should be told . . . Whatever decision is reached, there are two important factors. First, the patient should be told something. If it is not feasible to tell the patient his diagnosis and prognosis, enough information should be given the patient to allay his fear and gain his cooperation. The second important factor is that the doctor, nurse, patient's family, social service worker, minister, and other members of the health team, should know what information has been given to the patient. The nurse, in turn, will assume responsibility for giving necessary information to other members of the nursing team. Knowing what the patient has been told, the nurse is in a position to support and reinterpret the physician's plan of treatment.

HILKEMEYER, 1958, P. 123

RENILDA E. HILKEMEYER

CAREER PATH

Most of Renilda's classmates took private duty cases, the most common employment for graduate nurses at that time. Renilda took a couple of cases but really didn't enjoy this type of nursing. An opportunity came through the alumni office for her to go to St. Mary's Hospital in Jefferson City, MO, about 60 miles from her hometown, where they needed an operating room nurse. Although Renilda had little operating room experience, she decided to take the job. She was paid $50 a month, plus room and board, and lived in a building behind the hospital. She was assigned to scrub on her first day, her daily role for the scheduled 10–12 cases each day. Her supervisor, Sister Herman, greeted Renilda on her first morning by telling her, "Go pick out your instruments for the first case, sterilize them, and get started." Renilda explained her lack of experience but was told she was "just going to have to do it." Renilda heard Sister Herman say to the surgeon, "She don't know nothing!" Renilda was the only scrub nurse and was on continual call for emergencies. Despite rough beginnings, Sister Herman became a close friend to Renilda and her family.

About a year later, Renilda heard about nursing grants available through the Missouri Division of Health for public health nurses. Renilda completed the application, answering yes to having a car, when in truth she did not even know how to drive. She got the job, bought a car, and learned to drive. She began three years of covering 30 counties, ". . . doing district work even though [she] didn't know what it was in the beginning."

In 1940, Renilda became ill with pneumonia with pleural effusions and was diagnosed with tuberculosis. During the next few years, she received a variety of treatments. She stayed in a tuberculosis sanatorium for more than a year, where treatment consisted primarily of bed rest. Renilda was offered three alternative approaches to resting the lungs for healing: more bed rest, rib removal, or pneumoperitoneum treatment. She chose pneumoperitoneum treatment, which entailed pumping air into her stomach to raise her diaphragm so that her lungs could rest. When the air got low, the process was repeated. Renilda said that she felt as though she were pregnant. During her recovery, Renilda was not able to work, but through the Tuberculosis Rehabilitation Program, she completed her course work at George Peabody College for Teachers in Nashville, TN, for a bachelor's degree in nursing education. On recovery, Renilda served as Assistant Director at the General Hospital No. 1 School of Nursing in Kansas City, MO, from 1947–1949 and then became the assistant executive secretary for the Missouri State Nurses Association. During this period, 1949–1950, her interest in cancer nursing began to develop.

BUREAU OF CANCER CONTROL

In 1950, Renilda accepted a position as Consultant in Nursing Education in the Bureau of Cancer Control for the Missouri Division of Health in Jefferson City. In this role, she was assigned to the Ellis Fischel State Cancer Hospital to develop a program to teach cancer nursing to professionals. This 104-bed hospital in Columbia opened in 1940 and was owned and supported by the state of Missouri. Renilda had no administrative responsibilities within the hospital. She was, however, given broad responsibilities for implementing a program that would improve cancer care for patients in the hospital and community. She had to prepare public health and hospital-based nurses to improve patient teaching, upgrade the knowledge base of nursing school faculty, assist nurses to implement cancer care programs in their respective areas, and prepare care guidelines to better coordinate care across settings. This program is well described in a paper, "Teaching Cancer Nursing," published in *Nursing Outlook*. This major undertaking began at a time when no national network of cancer nurses, no specialty organization, and very few printed resources were available. The program was tremendously ambitious in its scope but also was highly successful under Renilda's enthusiastic leadership. She noted that she first had to learn all about cancer, its treatments, and patient care. Then she developed orientation programs, policies, and procedures for the care of patients at Ellis Fischel Cancer Center in Missouri. She developed a five-day continuing-education program that was used as a model in other locations. What began as a program for Ellis Fischel nurses soon became popular for nursing school faculty, other hospital nurses, and nurses from other cities and states. Few programs of this type were available anywhere in the country at that time.

During her time at Ellis Fischel, Renilda collaborated with others in promoting cancer nursing in organizations such as the American Cancer Society (ACS). Her first role in this organization was as a member of the Nursing Advisory Committee in 1954. She also held various offices during these years in the Missouri State Nurses Association, the Central Missouri League of Nursing, and the Missouri League for Nursing. In 1952, she began an eight-year term as a special consultant to the Nursing Section, Field Investigation, and Demonstration Branch of the National Cancer Institute's (NCI's) Department of Health, Education, and Welfare under the direction of Rosalie Peterson. These were years of developing professional networks, strengthening the visibility and contributions of nursing organizations, and giving unceasingly of her talents and ideas.

M.D. ANDERSON HOSPITAL AND TUMOR INSTITUTE

In 1955, Renilda was appointed the Director of Nursing at the newly opened (1954) M.D. Anderson Hospital and Tumor Institute, part of the University of Texas System Cancer Center.

Basically the program has embodied

1. An orientation program of one week for newly employed professional and auxiliary personnel.
2. A continuous inservice education program for professional and auxiliary nursing personnel.
3. A 5-day institute in cancer nursing for personnel of official and non official public health agencies, and faculty members from schools of nursing within and outside of the state.
4. Planned field visits by the consultant with the public health field staff.
5. Short- and long-term evaluation of the program by those taking part in it.
6. Development of better coordination between the Division of Health of Missouri and the Missouri Division of the American Cancer Society.

HILKEMEYER & KINNEY, 1956, P. 180

RENILDA E. HILKEMEYER

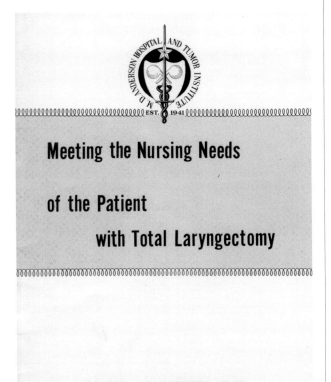

Meeting the Nursing Needs

of the Patient

with Total Laryngectomy

RENILDA HILKEMEYER, R. N.

DIRECTOR OF NURSING

ABOVE
A slide presentation used to educate nurses that was developed by Renilda Hilkemeyer

RIGHT
Renilda Hilkemeyer displaying supplies prior to demonstrating a procedure

She also held an academic appointment as professor in oncology nursing at the cancer center. Fewer than 200 nursing personnel were employed upon her arrival, but after her retirement, more than 1,000 nurses were on staff. She found some of the transition from Ellis Fischel to M.D. Anderson easy because she quickly saw that nurses had some of the same learning needs that she successfully had identified and met before. Although some needs were familiar, other challenges were new. Nurses at M.D. Anderson were in the forefront, working with other disciplines in expanded roles and innovative treatment approaches. Renilda noted that early nurse practice legislation made no provision for expanded roles. In Texas, the nurse's new status was not recognized until 1970. At that time, an amendment to the Nurse Practice Act for practitioners was passed.

It may be difficult to imagine the scope of care at this time and how few resources were available. Cancer care in the early years at M.D. Anderson focused on surgical care, in which patients often were treated without benefit of sophisticated anesthesia and anesthesia support, blood component therapy, and antibiotic therapy. Recovery rooms or surgical intensive care units were not available when the hospital was built, but both were added in the next few years. Nurses generally had only a very limited understanding of radiation therapy and radioisotope use. Renilda worked with the Radiation Protection Service and with physicians to develop quality care and protective policies and procedures. She noted in her recollections that few written materials were available on nursing care of this patient population. ACS distributed an article that she wrote in 1967 to nurses in other settings because of the lack of resource materials. In working with surgical patients, many challenges arose. The lack of disposable supplies for ostomy patients, for example, and the ineffectiveness of permanent appliances hampered patient recovery and quality of life. The administration of early chemotherapeutic agents and, later, biotherapeutic agents was not the role of the nurse. The care of the patient receiving them posed great challenges. Nurses began to develop new approaches for assessing and intervening in this care.

Early cancer nurses were generalists, and evidence of this is readily found in Renilda's writings. Few oncology nurses today could publish in areas as diverse as chemotherapy, radiation therapy, surgery, and nurs-

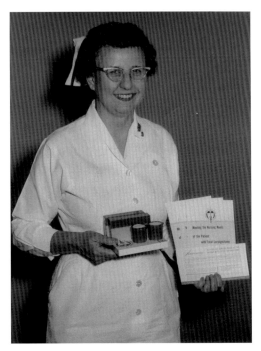

ing education, but Renilda's career spanned enough years for her to recognize the need for subspecialization. As early as 1974, Renilda made budget proposals to reorganize the nursing program to include clinical nurse specialists. Early budgets for this change were not approved, but, in 1978, the first three clinical nurse specialist positions were approved and filled.

Renilda took an active role in education not only for the M.D. Anderson nursing staff but for other nurses as well. In 1966, Renilda applied for a three-year grant from the Cancer Control Branch of the Division of Chronic Disease, Department of Health, Education, and Welfare. The program, "Preparation of Faculty and Administrative Nursing Personnel in Cancer Nursing," sought to improve the care of patients with cancer. Based on a strong belief that faculty and practice had to work together to make change, the program brought a faculty member and a nursing administrator from each participating school or facility. The teams came for five days to two weeks during a three-year period. Between sessions, assignments were given to provide application of the knowledge gained.

In 1972, Renilda had an initial meeting with Dr. John Bailar, associate director for Cancer Control at NCI. Unable to secure any time with Dr. Bailar because of his busy schedule, Renilda proposed her ideas for nursing education to him en route to the airport. She stressed her belief that established cancer centers should take leadership in the preparation of nurses to staff future cancer centers. Renilda followed up with a brief proposal outlining her ideas, a proposal that subsequently stimulated thinking about nursing education by NCI. In 1974, NCI issued a request for proposals for education programs that would encompass undergraduate, graduate, and continuing education. Renilda and the M.D. Anderson Cancer Hospital and Tumor Institute were awarded one of those contracts. This was the first of many connections between Renilda and NCI. From 1974–1984, she served as a consultant to the Special Projects Branch, and from 1979–1983, she was a member of the Cancer Control Grant Review Committee and a chairperson or member of site visit teams for NCI.

In professional nursing circles, Renilda was known as "Hilke." At M.D. Anderson, she always had been referred to as "Miss Hilkemeyer." During this time, this was probably an appropriate

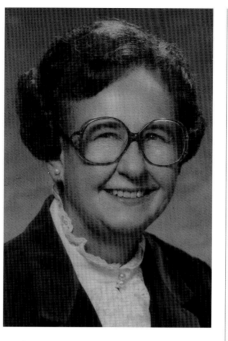

LEFT
Renilda Hilkemeyer

"Hilke" is a nurse to the core. She has high expectations and has always worked to ensure that nurses have the tools they need to give the finest care possible to their patients. At M.D. Anderson, Renilda worked hard to make sure that standards were high and that nurses had the education, technology, environment, leadership, and resources they needed to meet those standards. She also made sure that nurses were valued and that they received credit for the contributions they made to patient care. I came to M.D. Anderson because I needed a job. I stayed because, as an educator, I could see the value that was placed on the education of the staff. This is the legacy of Renilda Hilkemeyer.

BETTY CODY
UNIVERSITY OF TEXAS
M.D. ANDERSON CANCER CENTER

RENILDA E. HILKEMEYER

RIGHT
Program from first ACS National Conference on Cancer Nursing, 1973

BELOW
Renilda Hilkemeyer

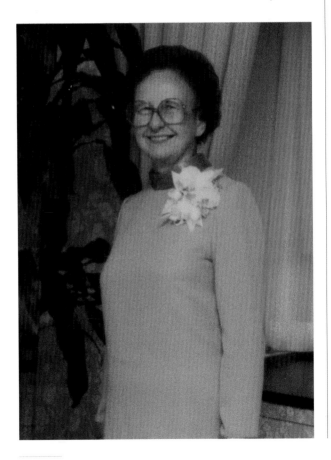

form of demonstrating respect. When people call her "Miss Hilkemeyer" today, it is used as a term of endearment.

During her early years at M.D. Anderson, Renilda met Virginia Barckley, the National Nursing Consultant for ACS. This was the beginning of a close professional and personal relationship that benefited both nurses and patients throughout the world. Virginia and Renilda frequently traveled together to present programs and used each other's knowledge and experience to develop program materials and propose ACS activities. In 1973, they worked with others to plan and carry out the first ACS National Conference on Cancer Nursing in Chicago. They were overwhelmed with the success of that meeting, which brought approximately 2,500 nurses together to focus on the differences they could make to patients with cancer.

Renilda served on ACS committees and made contributions to ACS that are too numerous to detail. One particularly memorable activity was when she and Virginia responded to a request by the World Health Organization to put on the First National Nursing Conference in Peru. "Of all the things we did together, the one we nearly croaked over was that trip to Peru," said Renilda. Arriving to find that none of the nurses spoke English, and not speaking Spanish themselves, they found an obstetrics nurse who could provide the translations of their content. Renilda and Virginia spent the night writing out their presentations so the content could be translated. These were not strictly podium presentations; they were practical demonstrations of equipment and procedures for which the American visitors improvised using any equipment they could find.

Renilda has held various ACS committee appointments for more than 45 years. Few nurses can boast of such a contribution. The committees and programs on which she served made many accomplishments. Of her many achievements, the crowning one has to be the establishment of the ACS Nursing Scholarship Program. Hundreds of oncology nurses have benefited from this program through funding for graduate and doctoral programs. No other nursing specialty has experienced this tremendous level of educational support from a national organization. The commitment of ACS to nurses over the decades clearly comes from the outstanding examples and hard work of

American Cancer Society's National Conference on Cancer Nursing

Program

dedicated leaders such as Renilda. ACS recognized her lifetime achievements through two of its highest awards, the ACS Distinguished Service Award and the National Nursing Leadership Award. ACS scholars and nursing school faculty members are living testaments to the goals envisioned by Renilda Hilkemeyer. Other awards she received included the Nurse of the Year Award in the Houston Area League for Nursing (1973) and the Texas Nurses Association Nurse of the Year Award (1979).

Another honor bestowed upon Renilda was the formation of the Renilda Hilkemeyer Child Care Center of the Texas Medical Center. Dr. R. Lee Clark, of M.D. Anderson, made the following remarks at the dedication ceremony of the center on October 12, 1981.

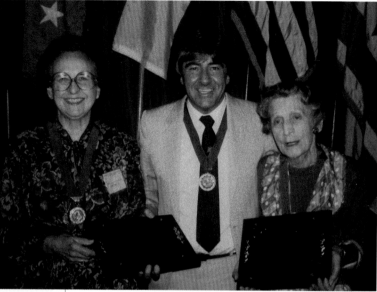

ABOVE
Renilda Hilkemeyer, Robert Tiffany, and Virginia Barckley receiving the International Society of Nurses in Cancer Care Distinguished Merit Award 1986

The lady we are honoring today . . . was one of the nurses interviewed for the position of Director of Nursing at the University of Texas M.D. Anderson Hospital and Tumor Institute—then only partially activated with 100 of its 300 beds, newly opened in February 1954. She got the job because of her demonstrated administrative and managerial ability, but especially for her devotion to the bedside care of the patient and her deep commitment to caring about and alleviating, if possible, much of the pathos and anxiety that is the lot of the cancer patient.

Miss Hilkemeyer is a luminous example of the steady, unremitting commitment to the daily alleviation of anxiety in its many forms. . . . This lady of whom we speak has a core of practicality, of realism, of efficiency as unshakable as that of any other outstanding general on any field of battle. But, she is the champion of women and children, well or ill, and of us men when we are weak and suffering or ignorant and willing to learn.

Allow me to "count" the ways she has translated her love into action.

- *She has instituted and supervised efficient and innovative nursing care for approximately 160,000 patients of M.D. Anderson Hospital since 1955.*
- *When our new Lutheran Pavilion Hospital was in the planning phase, she took the opportunity to request drastic redesigning of the traditional inpatient nursing station and patient rooms for maximum efficiency of routine and emergency care and for maximum communications interface between staff members and patients, thereby also alleviating anxiety induced by a feeling of isolation by distance.*

RENILDA E. HILKEMEYER

Any human being is potentially capable of feeling and expressing compassion. It seems to me, however, there is a qualitative difference in the way compassion is expressed by those who are in the health professions and deal directly with persons who are ill. This is particularly true of the nurse dealing with patients at the bedside. With her basic nurturing role in the earthly scheme, she quietly administers small steady doses of compassion and empathy by hour, by day, by year, even while she is solving problems. She seems to find gratification in solving the problems of how best to give solace and comfort than do many others.

R. LEE CLARK, MD
1981

- *She cosponsored, with the pediatric physicians, a nontraditional policy of making provisions for family members of pediatric patients to sleep overnight in the patients' rooms and to be able to use on-the-ward kitchen facilities for preparing favorite foods for their children.*
- *She solved the multifaceted problems of maintaining an adequate staff that could be less preoccupied with the problems of parenthood by working for the establishment of a Texas Medical Center Child Care Center, ensuring that the children of vital staff members could receive superior supervisory, medical, and educational care while their parents were pursuing the daily responsibilities to others.*
- *She has trained nursing personnel at Anderson to demonstrate their compassion as well as their nursing skills to patients and members of their families.*
- *She has instituted in-service training programs to keep nursing skills current and has made possible the opportunity for some personnel to seek training elsewhere when it was not available in Houston.*
- *She has sought and successfully acquired funds from every possible source to initiate and maintain programs.*
- *She has kept her nursing skills active, even though concentrating on administrative duties by attending patients when needed and with "private duty nursing" for family members and friends.*
- *Miss Hilkemeyer and her staff trained visiting nurses and other homecare personnel to administer supportive care to patients in their communities when those communities lacked the necessary services.*

She has [also] turned her intellect and energy toward the world. It must be evident to all that the primary reason M.D. Anderson Hospital and Tumor Institute is one of the renowned cancer centers in the world is because of Miss Hilkemeyer and other individuals of her stature, whose total dedication to service in every area of need lead them to higher and even higher levels of contribution. [Miss Hilkemeyer] has, by example and by encouragement, led thousands of young people into fulfillment of their benevolent and intellectual potential. What more fitting way to express our appreciation to this exceptional woman than by endowing a center dedicated to the nurturing of our future—our children—with her name.

R. LEE CLARK, MD
M.D. ANDERSON HOSPITAL
HOUSTON, TX

RETIREMENT

When Renilda retired from her last paid position, staff assistant to the president at the M.D. Anderson Hospital and Tumor Institute, it hardly meant the end of work for her. In fact, leaving her office may have been the only tangible sign of retirement. Renilda was serving as a member of the Surveillance Committee, the Institutional Review Board for the University of Texas Cancer Center, a post she had held since 1977 and continues to hold today. She also served in several ACS capacities at the time and completed terms in 1986 and 1987 on the Professional Education Committee and the National Advisory Committee, respectively. She went on to serve ACS through a one-year term on the Workstudy Group Task Force on Smoke Free Young America and was a consultant on a videotape production on cancer nursing through 1986. She has continued to be associated with the ACS Subcommittee on Scholarships and Professorships in Oncology Nursing.

Renilda always has been active in her church, and retirement from her regular work has afforded her an opportunity for more regular involvement. In 1985, she became a member as well as secretary of the Interfaith Hunger Coalition Advisory Council for the Houston Metropolitan Ministries. She has served as a volunteer at the Braes Interfaith Ministries (BIM) food pantry since 1985 and has been a member of its Board of Directors since 1990. She served as president of that board in 1990, 1991, 1994, and 1998. In 1997, she received the BIM Volunteer of the Year Award in recognition of more than 6,000 hours of faithful service rendered in meeting the needs of families and individuals in crisis.

SUMMARY

Summarizing the contributions of Renilda Hilkemeyer is difficult. Her resume attests to her many individual achievements. Her professional network included many nurses notable for their own contributions and who collectively began addressing the problem of caring for patients with cancer. Renilda and her colleagues appear to have been unshakable in their conviction that care could be improved and that nurses could be instrumental in this change. Convinced of their faith in each other, they went on to speak and write and share their knowledge. Renilda was visionary and convincing, and it is no surprise that she was one of four advisors chosen to form a society for oncology nurses, known as the Oncology Nursing Society. She had a wealth of experience from which to draw as this group began to look at the needs of nurses in cancer care and how these needs might be met.

Renilda is an excellent role model for nurses today. She welcomed challenge and made paths where none existed. Her zest for life and her love for people have marked her career and her life.

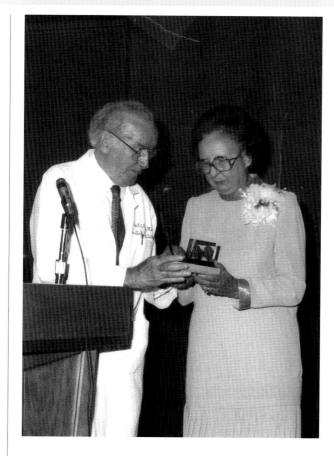

ABOVE
Robert E. Hickey honored Renilda upon her retirement with a pen with gold seals of the University of Texas System Cancer Center, M.D. Anderson Hospital and Tumor Institute. The inscription on it reads,

"In appreciation of your contribution to the progress of M.D. Anderson."

She remains keenly interested in cancer nursing and is vigorous in her applause for the progress nurses continue to make in this arena.

REFERENCES

Hilkemeyer, R. (1958). Nursing care of the cancer patient in the hospital and home. *Cancer: A Bulletin of Progress, 8*, 122–125.

Hilkemeyer, R. (1985). A historical perspective in cancer nursing. *Oncology Nursing Forum, 12*(1), 6–15.

Hilkemeyer, R. (1991). A glimpse into the past of cancer nursing. *Dimensions in Oncology Nursing, 5*(1), 5–8.

Hilkemeyer, R., & Kinney, H.E. (1956). Teaching cancer nursing. *Nursing Outlook, 4*(3), 177–180.

Honors come back to back for Renilda Hilkemeyer. (1981). *The University of Texas System Cancer Center Messenger, 10*(11), 1.

Zanca, J. (1993). Virginia Barckley: A lifetime of service, as told by her lifelong friend, Renilda Hilkemeyer. *Cancer Nursing News, 11*(4), 1–2.

Hilkemeyer, Renilda, interview by Susan Baird, 1987.

SELECTED WRITINGS
TEACHING CANCER NURSING (1956)

Nearly six years ago, an educational program in cancer nursing was initiated for professional and auxiliary personnel by the director of the Bureau of Nursing and the director of the Bureau of Cancer Control in the Division of Health of Missouri. It has a 4-fold purpose:

1. To assist the public health nurse to function more effectively in the cancer control program by broadening her background in cancer.
2. To better interpret and utilize an existing state facility, the Ellis Fischel State Cancer Hospital in Columbia, Missouri.
3. To assist in improving the nursing care of the cancer patient at this hospital.
4. To achieve better cooperation between the Bureau of Cancer Control in the Division of Health of Missouri and the Missouri Division of the American Cancer Society in coordinating the cancer control programs.

The Division of Health employed a consultant public health nurse to assist in implementing the program and assigned her to the Ellis Fischel State Cancer Hospital to serve in an advisory-educational capacity. She was given no administrative responsibilities within the hospital. She was, however, given the responsibility

1. To plan and take part in cancer nursing institutes at the Ellis Fischel State Cancer Hospital for the public health nursing staffs from both official and nonofficial agencies and for graduate nurse faculty members from schools of nursing.
2. To plan and take part in a program through which nurses in the hospital and public health nurses in the field might become more proficient in teaching patients.
3. To visit the public health staff in the field to give professional consultation in cancer nursing and related problems.
4. To assist in the preparation of guides and procedures to be used in both the hospital and the field so the care and teaching of patients would be coordinated.

Nursing Consultation Service

The basic plan of the nursing consultation service in the field is to visit each public health district each year and to make additional visits when requested. Before the consultant is scheduled to visit the field, she contacts the supervisor, who in turn finds out from the public health nurses in her area what their problems and needs are, and whether they want consultation service. From this information, the supervisor plans the schedule and notifies the consultant.

When the consultant goes into the field, she holds an initial conference with the supervisor to make the plans for the visit. If possible, the supervisor accompanies the consultant when she visits the field nurses so that she will know what they discuss. This ensures continued effective supervision and keeps the supervisor up to date. A final conference is held with the supervisor before the consultant leaves the field. Within a month of the field visit, the consultant sends a written report of it to the supervisor, to the director of the bureau of nursing, and to the director of the bureau of cancer control, if he wishes to have it.

Evaluation

Within two weeks after each public health nurse has completed the institute, she writes an evaluation for the director of the bureau of nursing. This is her immediate reaction to the learning experience and it is usually her impression of the hospital and its services, the staff and their relationship to the patient, the care that the patients receive, her increased knowledge of cancer, and the content of the program and how it was presented.

These evaluation reports indicate that the program has stimulated public health nurses to do more about cancer control and has helped them to visualize their potential contribution to cancer control programs. It has broadened their knowledge of the disease, enabling them to do more effective home visiting and education in their communities. It has helped them to interpret better the services and facilities of the cancer hospital and other community facilities for the care of the cancer patient. It has helped them to see the value of teaching the patient and to correlate the hospital's teaching with circumstances in the patient's home. It has shown them the value of follow-up service for the cancer patient and has enabled them to interpret this to patient, family, and community. Last, but certainly not least, it has changed their attitude toward cancer and the cancer patient. After the nurses have been in the field six months, a questionnaire is sent to them to see how they are using their educational experience in relation to themselves, their patients, and the community.

Summary

For the past six years, an educational program in cancer nursing has been carried on at the Ellis Fischel State Cancer Hospital in Columbia Missouri, by a consultant public health nurse from the state division of health who was assigned to the hospital.

References

1. Ellis Fischel State Cancer Hospital. *Annual Report*. Columbia, MO. July 1954.

2. Modlin, J. (1949). Five year results of cancer treatment at Ellis Fischel State Cancer Hospital; report to physician's of Missouri. *J Missouri MA, 46*, 485–488.
3. Hilkemeyer, R. (1951). The nursing education program at Ellis Fischel State Cancer Hospital. *Missouri Nurse*, April.

Biographical Statements

Miss Hilkemeyer (St. Louis University School of Nursing; BS George Peabody College for Teachers) as Consultant in Nursing Education with the Division of Health of Missouri was assigned to the Ellis Fischel Cancer Hospital to initiate and carry out the program described here. On September 1, 1955, she became director of nursing at the MD Anderson Hospital and Tumor Institute, University of Texas, Houston, TX.

Miss Kinney (Methodist, Brooklyn, NY; BS, MA, EdD Teachers College, Columbia University, NY) is director of the Bureau of Public Health Nursing of the Division of Health of Missouri. She developed the original idea for this program in cancer nursing and planned it with the director of the Bureau of Cancer Control.

Note. From "Teaching Cancer Nursing," by R. Hilkemeyer and H.E. Kinney, 1956, *Nursing Outlook, 4*(3), pp. 177–180. Copyright 1956 by Mosby, Inc. Excerpted with permission.

INTRA-ARTERIAL CANCER CHEMOTHERAPY (1966)

The Nurse's Responsibility in the Use of Investigational Drugs

With the increasing number of investigational and approved cancer chemotherapy drugs being made available, the professional nurse should be aware of her responsibility in the areas of preparation, administration, observation, nursing care of the patient, and recording . . .

The Role of the Nurse

What is the professional nurse's responsibility in giving cancer research drugs? The Code for Professional Nurses of the American Nurses' Association indicates her responsibility for her own acts based on her professional knowledge and judgment. The dependent nurse's function as described by the American Nurses' Association legal definition of nursing practice is "the administration of medications and treatments prescribed by the licensed physician and dentist." The nurse must have an understanding of the cause and effect of orders which she has carried out, and should question an order that is not clear. If she cannot clarify the order or does not have proper information, she should refuse to give the drug.

RENILDA E. HILKEMEYER

The professional nurse should be cognizant of the nursing practice act in the state in which she is practicing and she should be currently licensed to practice.

Professional nurses and state nurses' associations are concerned about the legal implications of professional practice in the area of dependent functions. Although medicine and nursing are recognized legally by statute as separate professions, there are "gray" areas of practice. State medical societies and state nurses' associations together with other official state agencies and hospital associations have formulated joint policy statements setting forth guide lines and criteria for professional nurse practice in specific areas. The professional nurse's responsibility in venipuncture and the administration of parenteral fluids has been officially defined by some states.

The American Hospital Association Board of Trustees issued in 1957 "A Statement of Principles Involved in the Use of Investigational Drugs in Hospitals." It was endorsed by the American Nurses' Association in 1962. These principles provide guide lines for the professional nurse and include requirements: (1) that investigational drugs be given only under the direct supervision of the principal investigator who has secured the necessary consent; (2) that research be conducted with adequate safety for the patient; (3) that when the nurse administers investigational drugs she should have basic information concerning the drug available to her; (4) that there be a central place where essential information about investigational drugs is available; and (5) that investigational drugs be stored in the pharmacy with provisions for proper labeling and dispensing on the physician investigator's written order. A Committee on Safety Practices and Procedures of the American Society of Hospital Pharmacists and a committee appointed by the Department of Hospital Nursing of the National League for Nursing met and published in November, 1959, "Proposed Safety Standards for Hospital Medication Procedures." Further work by this Committee resulted in a *Self-Evaluation Guide for Hospital Nursing Service Medication Safety.*

These guidelines can be used to establish and/or review standards for the professional nurse in administration of cancer chemotherapy investigational drugs.

The professional nurse in the hospital should know the policies and procedures relating to administration of cancer chemotherapy investigational drugs as established by nursing, hospital administration and the medical staff.

Note. From "Intra-arterial Chemotherapy," by R. Hilkemeyer, 1966, *Nursing Clinics of North America, 1*(2), pp. 295–307. Copyright 1966 by W. B. Saunders Company. Excerpted with permission.

TRIBUTES

If you are a pioneer, you are considered the "old guard" regardless of your age. Labeling, however, has never been a deterrent for Renilda. In 1975, when the Oncology Nursing Society was founded, the officers were considered so young that a "more seasoned advisory board" was appointed. Renilda was one of the appointees, and now she chuckles, "They never paid any attention to us. They just did what they wanted to do and that was fine with us." The appointment itself personifies the esteem she is afforded in the ranks of oncology nursing.

Renilda's acclaim always has extended beyond nursing; however, on many occasions, she used the multidisciplinary respect she earned to achieve the goals of the nursing profession. Having established herself and M.D. Anderson in oncology nursing long before the advent of formal oncology nursing education and educational resources, she vowed to make a difference for those who followed. When she arrived at M.D. Anderson, her first job was to convince some of the medical staff that nursing was different from medicine and that each made a unique contribution to cancer care. Evidently she was successful, because when Renilda subsequently served on various boards with the elite core of oncologists launched by M.D. Anderson, they listened when she spoke.

Renilda had a way of working with key individuals to gain support before springing new ideas on a formal board or committee. She always did her homework, garnered her resources, and anticipated the counter arguments. Then she patiently worked her miracles, achieving the unthinkable.

The respect for Renilda's proposals was exemplified most graphically by responses to her efforts to establish American Cancer Society (ACS) scholarships and professorships. When she proposed master's level scholarships in 1958, the first response was, "We can't do that. We haven't provided scholarships for any of the other professions, and that would just open the floodgates." Renilda was not deterred. She proceeded to convince members of the board that irrespective of the needs of other professions, the support of oncology nursing education was an important priority in cancer care. How did she do this? She did it systematically. Armed with a valid, well-documented argument, she gained an audience with selected colleagues who had witnessed the difference nursing at M.D. Anderson made for patients. She even was known to target individuals who were married to nurses, thus garnering an informed audience who could convince the uninformed.

I often had the privilege of being with Renilda before appointments with key individuals. She was driven by the gravity of her mission. In each approach, she selected an informed, influential nursing colleague to accompany her. Unknowingly, she was tutoring "the younger generation" even as she set and achieved goals. The success of her missions was predictable, although often painfully slow. Again, she was teaching younger colleagues to persevere. ACS nursing scholarships

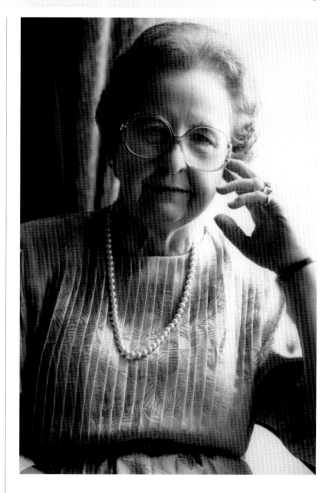

ABOVE
Renilda Hilkemeyer

RENILDA E. HILKEMEYER

were approved in principle in 1958, but they were not funded until 1980. Who other than Renilda would have persevered for so long?

Did she stop there? You know the answer. The initial amount of funding proposed for masters' in nursing scholarships was meager and unacceptable to Renilda because it failed to meet the goal of facilitating full-time study. The amount was increased. In 1981, 10 scholarships were funded, and on the insistence of the nursing committee, the number of students funded the following year was increased to 20.

Having achieved that goal, Renilda insisted that, "we need qualified faculty and researchers to ensure the quality of the master's programs and patient research." In 1986, doctoral scholarships for nurses were approved and simultaneously funded. Board members who opposed her proposal later noted that after Renilda's erudite argument for funding, they would rather have voted against motherhood than oppose her motion.

As strides were made in gaining support for oncology nursing education, Renilda was working equally as hard at establishing a process that ensured the selection of the best qualified and most highly committed applicants. The floodgates opened in the first years the scholarships were offered. Appointment to the ACS Scholarship Review Committee conferred the privilege of spending hours plowing through hundreds of long, detailed applications. Committee members independently ranked each applicant on stated criteria, then attended a two-day grueling meeting in New York at which group consensus on rankings was achieved. Annual reports were required and reviewed by the committee as well.

In 1980, the ACS nursing education program was expanded further to include the funding of professorships. Again, this program was not static. The number of professorships was increased as state divisions joined the ranks of sponsoring agencies. Reporting procedures became more stringent, with the Nursing Committee making site visits before approving each professorship. Renilda's wisdom surfaced in her insistence on meeting with the dean of nursing to ensure support from the university. Thus, site visitors became advocates for the professor. The Nursing Committee reviewed annual reports, and site visits were arranged if problems arose with the achievement of stated objectives. Under Renilda's tutelage, the nursing scholarship and professorship program became a model that ACS used to require goal delineation and systematic evaluation in other professional groups.

Rose F. McGee, RN, PhD

Professor of Nursing
Emory University

I first met Ms. Hilkemeyer in 1970 when I was hired as a nurse at M.D. Anderson. As Chief Nurse Executive, she was confident, knowledgeable, respected, and in control. During the next 20 years, while working under her command, I became more and more impressed with Renilda's determination to build a world-class nursing department. She was fair and encouraged innovations, but most of all, she expected nothing but the best in quality of patient care. Ms. Hilkemeyer is truly a legend in oncology nursing and executive leadership. I am very fortunate to have had the privilege of working with her during the past 30 years.

Cecil Brewer

Clinical Administrative Director
Ambulatory Treatment Center
University of Texas
M.D. Anderson Cancer Center

Renilda Hilkemeyer paved the way for me in many areas, encouraging me to seek administrative positions and recommending that I submit my name for the Texas Nurses Association ballot for election to the CEARP committee. I won that election and served on the committee as co-chairman for three years. She also encouraged me to become a delegate to the American Nurses Association convention in 1974, at which I represented the state of Texas.

Renilda was always an advocate for the staff, smiling in the face of adversity, and her hearty laugh has defused many tense situations. She has committed her life to oncology nursing, and it is a privilege to consider her my greatest mentor and a close friend.

Gary Houston

Former Director of Nursing
University of Texas
M.D. Anderson Cancer Center

Renilda Hilkemeyer always thought of "her" nurses first. She made sure that nursing staff knew what was going on in the institution and that we were well represented within the institution and in its numerous efforts.

My first memory of Renilda is from when I was a nursing student working at the world-famous M.D. Anderson Hospital and Tumor Institute. My paycheck for two shifts of 11–7 weekend work did not get processed, and I had no check to pick up on my way out of town to Mardis Gras in New Orleans. Ms. Hilkemeyer heard me complaining bitterly to the payroll staff and came out of her office and offered to write me a personal check to cover what I was owed. Needless to say, I left the office embarrassed to have made such a fool of myself!

Ms. Hilkemeyer also always supported the nursing staff in our efforts to continue work toward BSN and MS degrees. She facilitated flexible work hours so that we could attend school and hold full-time positions. Today, many of the staff members at M.D. Anderson hold their positions because of her encouragement to continue their education as well as to try new and different types of work assignments. Renilda Hilkemeyer had a tremendous impact on my life, and to this day, I consider her a dear friend and mentor.

Debbie Houston
Associate Director
Management Information Systems
University of Texas
M.D. Anderson Cancer Center

There are a few things I remember about Hilke.

She always had a messy desk, but whenever she needed something, it was immediately under her fingers; she was very organized about her work.

She was impassioned about nurses knowing what they were doing, and it was equally important that the patients knew how to care for themselves. She encouraged new ideas and innovative care measures for the best treatment of our patients (the Alzet osmotic pump was a prototype of ambulatory treatment pumps and was tested at M.D. Anderson by one of the nurses).

She believed in nurses being a part of clinical research review (medical protocols). She served on this committee first as a nurse and now as a consumer.

Mary Ann Gilmore
Advanced Practice Nurse
University of Texas
M.D. Anderson Cancer Center

Professional papers and effects of Renilda Hilkemeyer are located in the archives at the National Office of the Oncology Nursing Society in Pittsburgh, PA.

JOSEPHINE K. CRAYTOR, RN, MS, FAAN
Leader in Cancer Nursing Education and Development of Nurse-Physician Collaborative Practice

"A clinic can be an educational center for student nurses, with opportunities for teaching and learning through a free interchange of ideas."

—*Josephine K. Craytor*

JOSEPHINE K. CRAYTOR

SIGNIFICANT CAREER CONTRIBUTIONS

- Held a joint faculty position at the University of Rochester in New York from 1960–1978 that comprised both clinical practice and teaching

- Developed, in conjunction with Dr. Charles Sherman and Dr. E. Savlov, the first Chemotherapy Clinic at Strong Memorial Hospital in Rochester

- Codirected, with Dr. Sherman, a demonstration project in "Team Care of Cancer Patients," which led to student nurses gaining cancer nursing experience in an outpatient setting

- Pioneered the role of the unification model of practice and the master's-prepared clinical nurse specialist

- Coauthored *The Nurse and the Cancer Patient: A Programmed Text,* which was widely used in nursing schools to teach cancer content

- Founded a nursing tract with cancer nursing as a specialty in the graduate program at the University of Rochester School of Nursing in New York

BIOGRAPHICAL INFORMATION

BIRTH

Josephine (Jo) Huston Kelly was born on October 30, 1915, in Xenia, OH.

PARENTS

Jo's father, James Kelly, was born in Xenia, OH, in 1885. His ancestry dates back to pre-Revolutionary America. His great-grandfather was the first of his family to emigrate from Ireland. He settled in Ohio and founded a cordage mill, the first of its kind west of the Appalachian Mountains. The mill was a successful family business for many years. James and his brother inherited the mill and later sold it in 1929, shortly before the Depression. James' interest in sports was evident through his acquisition of a sporting goods store and a professional girls' basketball team, both in Ohio. After moving to Florida, he acquired two hunting lodges. Jo's father died from pneumonia in 1963.

Jo's mother, Isabel Damon Whitmore, was born in 1888. She had an artistic background; she trained in voice, painted, and did original embroidery work. James and Isabel married in Ohio in 1910. Isabel gave birth to their first child, Josephine, in 1915, followed by the birth of two more girls.

They moved several times during their marriage, living in Ohio, North Carolina, and Florida. When Jo was 10 years old, her parents divorced. At first, Isabel and her daughters remained in Xenia, living first with her parents and then with her brother in Antioch. Later, they moved to North Carolina, where Isabel enjoyed the warm winters and riding horses. However, family ties brought the women back to Ohio. The girls attended various schools, both public and private, and, upon reaching high school, lived at a boarding school in North Carolina. Isabel developed breast cancer and died at age 56.

FAMILY

Jo was the oldest of three daughters. Her sister, Barbara, who was just one year younger, went to Florida following high school to help her father run his hunting lodges. She married and had two children. Barbara, like her mother, died of breast cancer around the age of 50. Virginia, who was six years younger then Jo, graduated from Radcliff College in fine arts and attended New York University on an engineering scholarship. In the early 1950s, Virginia was diagnosed with a life-threatening brain tumor, which was surgically removed. Although the tumor was benign, it caused some temporary paralysis and loss of speech. In spite of this, Virginia later became an accomplished interior designer in New York City.

Jo recalls her childhood as being interesting and stimulating, filled with books, art classes, and music lessons. However, she experienced some periods of loneliness because the family was never settled in any one place for long. After boarding school in North Carolina, Jo returned to Ohio, and, in 1933, she entered the Western College for Women in Oxford, OH. She was deeply involved in school activities, was president of the freshman class, and worked in the chemistry laboratory to earn money for school. Jo's grandmother helped her to pay for room and board. The college faculty was mostly women, who subtly conveyed the message that girls are as capable and important as boys. This message, along with the influence of a roommate's family with whom she spent Christmas holidays, provided the turning point in Jo's career choice. Her roommate's father was a physician, her mother a nurse, and her cousin a senior medical student. They exposed her to medicine as a career, something she had not considered previously.

During the Depression, it became financially impossible for Jo to continue college. She decided to go into nursing, a choice her family did not favor because they viewed nursing as equal to that of becoming a domestic servant. The director of a coeducational camp at a New York City settlement house, where Jo had worked during the summers, urged her to apply to the New York Hospital School of Nursing at Cornell University. Jo found the school challenging with its high academic standards, excellent faculty, and superb clinical opportunities. In 1938, Jo received her diploma in nursing.

CAREER PATH

Jo had her first article published, while still a nursing student, in the *American Journal of Nursing* in 1938. She wrote about the psychological needs of the gynecological patient and the role that nurses could play in helping patients to get the recognition they deserve. Even as a student, Jo recognized the need to see beyond the "patient in the bed." In a second article, published in 1941, Jo called for an interchange of ideas and cooperation between the parents of the ill child and members of the healthcare team. Specifically, Jo viewed the pediatric clinic as an educational center, with numerous learning opportunities for parents and student nurses.

For the first two years following graduation, Jo combined working in the Children's Clinic in the New York Hospital with night school at Teachers College at Columbia University. Jo met and married Russell Craytor during her days as a student nurse. At the time, Russ recently had graduated from college and was working in New York City for an optical company, Bausch and Lomb. In 1942, Jo stepped away from her professional career in exchange for the role of wife and mother to their

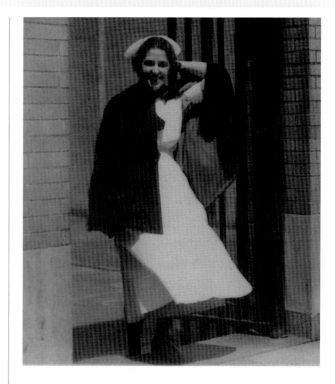

ABOVE
Josephine Kelly
Cornell University
New York Hospital
School of Nursing
1938

"The doctor cures the physical ills of the patient (with the nurse's aid) but it is up to the nurse to help that patient to become a person once more able to face and cope with life. The task is a responsibility and a privilege."

KELLY, 1938, P. 472

JOSEPHINE K. CRAYTOR

RIGHT
Josephine Craytor holding her
daughter Barbara
1943

BELOW
Josephine Craytor
Associate Professor and Director of
the course Introduction to Nursing
University of Rochester
School of Nursing
1959

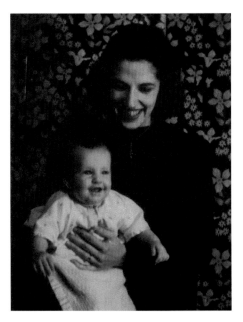

RIGHT
Josephine Craytor holding her
daughter Barbara
1943

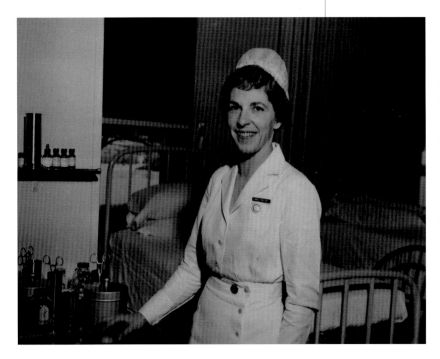

first born, Barbara. Following the bombing of Pearl Harbor, Russ was called to work at the Bausch and Lomb plant in Rochester, NY. Jo took advantage of being close to the University of Rochester and attended night school, completing a bachelor's degree in general studies in 1946. She had a distinguished academic record and was elected to Phi Beta Kappa, an honors society. Her graduation coincided with her husband's appointment to direct the Bausch and Lomb offices in New York City and the birth of their second daughter, Wendy. The Craytor family moved back to Rochester in 1948, and this time Russ's position at the Rochester Bausch and Lomb plant was to be permanent. Jo had experienced several miscarriages and lost one child, who was born premature. After 16 years of being devoted to her home, husband, and two daughters, Jo decided to return to work.

UNIVERSITY OF ROCHESTER

Eleanor Hall, the dean at the University of Rochester School of Nursing, offered Jo a faculty position. Her first teaching responsibility was to develop and implement a new course, Fundamentals of Nursing, for students in the three-year diploma and five-year degree programs. Jo taught that the social and emotional needs of patients need to be considered along with their physiological needs and that students need to believe in the importance of what they, as nurses, have to contribute to patient care.

From 1959–1960, Jo took an educational leave from teaching to complete her master's degree in science with a major in nursing education. For her thesis, she chose to develop and demonstrate a role for the master's-prepared nurse on the health team as a co-worker to a physician. This was a bold step to take in 1960 and later laid the groundwork for the role of a clinical nurse specialist. Jo chose this undertaking because she felt that communication between the nurse and physician pertaining to patient care was very limited. Reports in the popular press claimed that nurses had become scientific and had no compassion. Colleagues thought her project was crazy and told her that they would not dare try such a presumptuous idea. Physicians expected her to do the traditional nursing activities such as setting up dressings and preparing the patient for an examination. She found herself defining the nursing needs of a patient to a team of skeptical doctors, and her questions, which were meant to clarify nursing responsibilities, were perceived as a challenge to physicians' plans for medical care. Jo created a tentative operational definition of the job of a nurse on the health team and gathered reactions of nurses and physicians to this document. Her findings were compiled as part of her thesis, "An Action Research Project: An Experimental Physician-Nurse Approach to Patient Care."

A TENTATIVE OPERATIONAL DEFINITION OF THE JOB OF A NURSE ON THE HEALTH TEAM

This definition was developed for use in a particular medical center setting with a team made up of an attending physician, his resident staff, and a team nurse.

1. The team nurse is a graduate nurse who works directly with the physician and his resident staff in the care of this physician's patients wherever they may be in the hospital.

2. The team nurse participates with the medical team in planning care for the patients involved by trying to define those aspects of care which are nursing, and by suggesting nursing measures appropriate to the medical plan of care and the needs of the patient.

3. The team nurse assists the physician in planning medical care by bringing together her own observations, those of the personnel on the patient's unit, and those of other paramedical personnel, of the condition of the patient, his response to treatment and individual preferences or problems which may affect care or recovery.

4. The team nurse helps the patient and his family to understand and accept his condition and treatment by amplifying the physician's explanations and by explaining methods of treatment.

5. The team nurse interprets, to whatever extent seems necessary, the medical plan of care to the floor nursing personnel, and works with them in developing appropriate nursing care plans for the patient. She can review the patient's history, the present treatment regimen and, in-so-far as she is able, the rationale governing treatment.

6. With the help of all personnel involved in the care of the patient the team nurse determines the patient's need for teaching of measures of self-care in the hospital and in preparation for discharge from the hospital. She involves the patient's family in this teaching to whatever extent seems desirable. She can teach the patient herself, help the floor personnel in this, or help in supplying information for referrals to cooperating agencies.

7. The team nurse does whatever reading and investigation seems necessary to increase her knowledge of the nursing problems presented by the patient so that she can help the floor personnel increase their knowledge and modify care methods to meet the needs of the patient.

8. The team nurse attempts to coordinate the care of the patient by face-to-face discussion of his condition, his needs as observed, and the over-all medical plans with other paramedical personnel involved in his care. (Soc. Service, Dietetics, Physical Therapy, etc.)

(continued on next page)

9. The team nurse consults whatever resources are available (with the approval of the physician) to learn more about the patient when special problems present themselves. Socio-economic problems are handled by the social worker with input from the team nurse and with communication back to the team nurse.

10. The team nurse records in Nurses' Notes pertinent material about specific nursing care plans, teaching done or progress in some form of treatment not otherwise recorded.

11. The team nurse develops whatever methods of communication seem most helpful, with the medical team, the floor nursing personnel and others involved in care. She participates as asked in nursing team conferences and class sessions.

At no time should the team nurse interfere with established methods of communications or offer gratuitous advice about care of patients, unless patient safety appears to be endangered. Her role is to help and reinforce what is being done, to bring new information for consideration and to encourage creativity in planning and giving care. If elements of care which seem important to the team nurse are weak or lacking she can give the care herself or help in seeing that it is given.

JOSEPHINE K. CRAYTOR
ROCHESTER, NEW YORK
NOVEMBER 1959

Gradually, Jo was accepted as a team member and valued for her contribution in planning care for the patient. The unification model of practice arose from this pioneering work.

After obtaining her master's degree, Jo returned to the University of Rochester School of Nursing to teach medical-surgical nursing and to develop a demonstration project in "Team Care of Cancer Patients" with Dr. Charles Sherman. The grant was funded for a three-year period and Jo, in conjunction with her faculty position, assumed the nurse's role on the cancer project. Her work consisted of teaching and committee obligations in the nursing department, attendance at tumor rounds and resident's rounds in radiation therapy, carrying her own caseload of referred patients, serving as the Medical Center nursing consultant on problems of cancer nursing, and the role of administrator of the Tumor Clinics. In 1962, she collaborated with Dr. Sherman and Dr. E. Savlov in setting up the first chemotherapy outpatient clinic. Her strategies for integrating the clinical setting with education included bringing patients to class and conferences, inviting former patients to visit new patients who had mastectomies and colostomies, and having student nurses in clinical rounds and conferences. Jo believed in teaching by doing. She was a role model for students in the clinical setting, as well as in the classroom, at a time when a nursing instructor was very separate from a practitioner.

Jo's interest in facilitating independent learning fueled her predilection in programmed learning, the development of a teaching program for nurses in radiation therapy, and a textbook using a programmed format, *The Nurse and the Cancer Patient: A Programmed Text*. Her reputation and expertise in this approach to learning led to her success in acquiring grants from the Division of Nursing to conduct summer workshops in programming for self-instruction in nursing. Nurses from across the country attended these workshops.

When the graduate program in nursing at the University of Rochester moved to the School of Nursing, Jo took over the clinical courses and had students identify a nursing specialty that fostered their in-depth learning in one specific area of nursing. This innovation represents the educational pioneering of the master's-prepared clinical nurse specialist. From this emerged an oncology nursing tract and what is known today as the master's-prepared oncology clinical nurse specialist. Throughout her tenure, Jo's role consistently integrated education and clinical practice in carrying out her faculty responsibilities. When the Regional Medical Program was initiated at Strong Memorial Hospital, she was identified as the cancer nursing specialist, teaching many continuing-education courses. In 1975, Jo was named the first Associate Director for Oncology Nursing at the university's Cancer Center.

By the mid-1960s, Jo was considered an expert in cancer nursing not only at the University of Rochester but also throughout the country. Within New York, she participated in numerous Cancer Teaching Days and was the only nurse appointed to the governor's 1976 Ad Hoc Committee on Early Detection of Breast Cancer. At the national level, Jo was invited to serve on the Nursing Advisory Board of the American Cancer Society (ACS), as a faculty member for national conferences on cancer nursing, as consultant at the National Cancer Institute's (NCI's) Division of Resources, Centers, and Community Resources, and as the first nurse member of the American Association for Cancer Education.

RETIREMENT

In 1978, Jo retired after 21 years at the University of Rochester. The university bestowed her the title of Professor Emeritus. After retirement, she participated in school activities as a board member of the Deans Advisory Committee, was active in fund-raising for the school, and was a member of the Trustees' Council. Jo also took an active role in the Friends of Strong

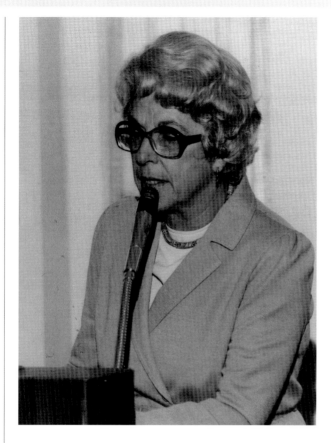

ABOVE
Josephine Craytor
1979

JOSEPHINE K. CRAYTOR

RIGHT
Josephine Craytor
Radiation therapy volunteer
1988

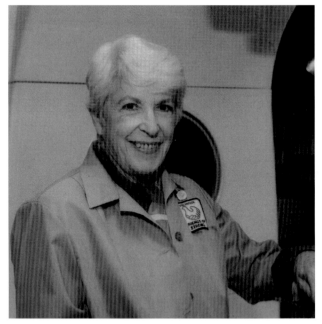

CHARLES D. SHERMAN, JR., M. D.
WESTFALL PARK MEDICAL CENTER
2253 CLINTON AVENUE SOUTH
ROCHESTER, NEW YORK 14610
—
TELEPHONE 473-7172 (WESTFALL)

STRONG MEMORIAL OFFICE 275-2755
CANCER CHEMOTHERAPY 275-5500

September 14, 1973

Mrs. Nancy Dainty
R.D. #3 County Road 33
Canandaigua, New York 14424

RE: Mrs. Josephine Craytor

Dear Mrs. Dainty:

I have known Mrs. Craytor for 20 years and have worked with her ever since she first came to the University in the late 50's. She has an exceptional ability to work with physicians, students, patients and others and the facility to arrive at the best possible outcome in any given situation involving various groups. She is highly intelligent and industrious and has made many contributions at the local, state and national level to the fields of cancer care and cancer nursing. I assume that you have her curriculum vitae and will not try to ennumerate her large number of accommplishments these last 15 years.

I can think of no one on the nursing faculty who would be more qualified to receive an alumni citation than Mrs. Craytor.

Sincerely yours,

Charles D. Sherman, Jr., M.D.
Clinical Professor of Surgery
University of Rochester
Medical Center

CDS:ac

Memorial Hospital and used her expertise to build a bridge between nursing in the clinical setting and hospital volunteers. She also organized the university's annual career day and would take groups on tours of the hospital. Her professional contributions to cancer nursing have continued as well. She has served as a consultant to the Clinical Cancer Education Program of NCI, was invited to participate in the International Union Against Cancer's first nursing sessions held during their 1978 Congress in Argentina and at the Asian Cancer Congress in India, has served on a community health hospice board, was a member of the archives committee of the Oncology Nursing Society (ONS), and was a member of the editorial board of *Cancer Nursing*.

Jo has received numerous awards for scholarship, teaching, and service. The New York State Nurses Association inducted her into its Society of Distinguished Practitioners in 1973, and, the following year, she became a fellow in the American Academy of Nursing. The University of Rochester presented her with the Alumni Award to Faculty, Distinguished Alumnus Award, Curtis Award for Excellence in Undergraduate Teaching, and Honorary Life Membership in the Alumni Association. ACS recognized Jo with its Distinguished Nursing Award and its Distinguished Service Award. She also has been honored as the first recipient of the Gittilmen Award to a Health Professional for Distinguished Service in Cancer Care and was the first Honorary Life Member of ONS.

Jo and her husband, Russ, moved from their home to a retirement community in the Rochester area. Their daughter, Barbara, graduated from Western Michigan University in home economics and currently lives in Florida with her husband. Her three children provide Jo and Russ with the delights of grandparenthood. Wendy received her bachelor's degree from the University of Rochester in psychology and completed a master's degree in business administration and healthcare planning at the University of Hawaii.

Retirement has provided Jo and Russ with the time and freedom to do what they love best—traveling and playing golf and bridge. They have traveled extensively throughout the world, with only two countries that they still would like to visit: Australia and Mexico. Jo recently had a mastectomy for early-stage breast cancer, and both she and Russ have pacemakers. They view these medical problems as inconveniences and minor setbacks to enjoying an active life. Jo spends one morning a week at a ceramics class, which is evident by the array of pottery dishes and artwork displayed in her home. She is also a member of the History Class, which is a group of women who attended eastern colleges. This club was created in 1890 and has been active ever since. The group meets six to seven times a year, at which time a member will present a historic paper on a person or topic that she has researched. The presentations are followed by a tea party and social time. Currently, 23 women belong to the organization, and new members must be under the age of 50. Jo finds this group of women very interesting and mentally stimulating. She and Russ now divide their time among their apartment, a cottage near the Finger Lake region of New York, and visits to their daughters in Florida and Alaska.

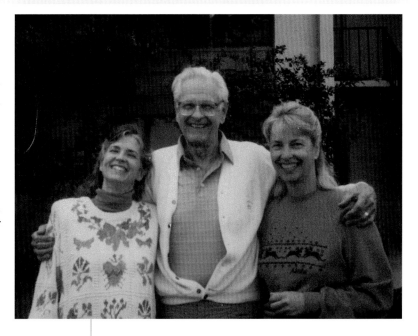

ABOVE
Josephine Craytor's husband
Russell and daughters, Wendy (left)
and Barbara (right)
1990

SUMMARY

Jo's leadership in oncology nursing has made an impact on the quality of life for many people with cancer and their family members. She exemplifies the attributes of an excellent teacher. She was an expert clinician who continually sought knowledge to improve her own professional competence. In reflecting over her professional career, her earliest pioneering efforts involved changing relationships between the nurse and the individual patient and the nurse and the physician, constant efforts to better understand the reactions of patients to their problems, and efforts to broaden the scope of nursing interventions. Through her practice as teacher and clinician, she contributed to new understandings of the potential of professional nursing. In the words of Loretta Ford, RN, EdD, dean at the University of Rochester School of Nursing, "In her many roles as consultant, educator, author, administrator, and practitioner, she has become a prophet in her own land—and in other lands as well." Oncology nurses have been the benefactors of Jo Craytor's many successful endeavors.

REFERENCES

Craytor, J.K. (1941). Teaching in the pediatric clinic. *Public Health Nursing, 33*, 666–670.

Craytor, J.K. (1959). *Journal of a risk-taker: Notes from a pioneer in cancer nursing.* Personal records kept by Josephine Craytor.

Craytor, J.K. (1960). *Developing a definition of the job of the nurse on the health team.* Personal papers from graduate school, University of Rochester, NY.

Craytor, J.K. (1985). Highlights in education for cancer nursing [Review]. *Oncology Nursing Forum, 12*(Suppl. 1), 19–27.

Kelly, J. (1938). Some psychological aspects of gynecological nursing. *American Journal of Nursing, 38*, 470–472.

University of Rochester School of Nursing. (1984). Alumni profile: Meet Josephine Craytor. *Pulse, 14*(3), 1–4.

Craytor, Josephine, interview by Nancy Hare, Oral History, University of Rochester School of Nursing, October 1994.

Craytor, Josephine, and colleagues from the University of Rochester School of Nursing, interview by Judith Johnson, April 1999.

SELECTED WRITINGS

ASSESSING LEARNING NEEDS OF NURSES WHO CARE FOR PERSONS WITH CANCER (1978)

Abstract: A series of three studies were carried out to determine nurses' needs for continuing education in cancer, identify nurses' perceptions of cancer patients and nurses, and test an educational intervention to upgrade skills and enhance satisfaction. In the first study, a stratified sample of 187 nurses in 10 counties separated more important from less important patient problems, identified learning needs, and differentiated among successful nursing interventions. In the second study, 100 nurses in an acute general hospital made decisions similar to the first group and reported perceptions of cancer patients as compared to typical hospital patients and of themselves as compared to the nurse best suited to cancer care. The third study tested an educational intervention based on individual needs and showed change in nurses' perceptions of cancer patients and of themselves, suggesting movement toward less stereotyping of patients and feelings of more competence among nurses.

The objectives of these studies were 1) to develop continuing education programs that would capitalize on nurses' readiness to learn and 2) to design and implement staff development programs which would increase nurses' involvement in cancer care and ultimately improve the quality of that care by upgrading nurses' skills and increasing the degree of satisfaction from their work with cancer patients.

All groups indicated a need to keep up with current therapy for cancer and the nursing measures necessary to help patients tolerate therapy. In addition, a high percentage of the respondents felt that helping patients deal with the emotional and psychological issues related to their illness, working with families, and dealing with their own feelings about cancer are not managed as well as they might be. Nurses in the quasi-experimental study responded in a very positive way to the individual attention, the opportunity to express negative feelings, and the positive reinforcement of successful practices. Of interest was the fact that after completion of the study, a number of the staff requested that their unit be designated as a specialized oncology division.

During the course of these studies, a process and techniques useful in defining nurses' needs for continuing education in cancer care were developed. Based on the defined needs, an educational intervention was planned and the usefulness of such a program was demonstrated. The process, or parts of it, may be appropriate for use in many health-care settings where nurses face challenging demands.

Note. From "Assessing Learning Needs of Nurses Who Care for Persons With Cancer," by J.K. Craytor, J.K. Brown, and G.R. Morrow, 1978, *Cancer Nursing*, *1*, pp. 211–220. Copyright 1978 by Lippincott Williams and Wilkins. Excerpted with permission.

TALKING WITH PERSONS WHO HAVE CANCER (1969)
Ways With Words

Nurses use talk in several ways. First, it provides for the exchange of information—explanations, instructions, fact-gathering, planning, and teaching. Second, talking is an indispensable therapeutic tool to relieve anxiety and increase comfort, which is the very heart of nursing.

Third, talking is used to fill time. It can divert or amuse a patient when he is so anxious that he must have time to structure his situation.

Meaningful verbal communication is far more than an exchange of words. It is an exchange of understood meanings. If a patient is to comprehend the message, he must hear what is said and understand the words which are used. Explanations need to be clear and uncomplicated. Only by getting feedback, evidence that the message was or was not received, can the nurse be sure that the patient heard what she said. The most direct way to get feedback is to ask the patient what he understands.

An incident in a dermatology clinic illustrates the importance of feedback. An elderly woman returned to the clinic for a report. A lesion on her nose had been biopsied the week before. The nurse heard the physician explain that the lesion was a small skin cancer of a relatively harmless type that does not spread and that it had been completely removed. Later the nurse noticed the woman sitting apathetically in the waiting room. "You look sad," she said. "What is the trouble?"

The patient responded, "I guess I'm going to die." The nurse asked, "What makes you think that?" "I have cancer," the woman replied. The patient had heard part of the message. Had the nurse not sought feedback she might not have known that this woman needed to talk about cancer or needed clarification of the doctor's explanation.

It is also important for the nurse to indicate that she understands what the patient is trying to tell her. She can acknowledge his message by stating what she thinks she heard, and asking if she is correct.

. . . most patients use talk for interpersonal contact as well as to get information. Meaningful communication reduces the feeling of loneliness and isolation, which is usually part of illness. Since the pressure of tasks and the rapid turnover of patients and staff in an acute-care hospital reduce the number and length of contacts between a patient and any given nurse, making each contact helpful is important.

Uneasy Feelings

The way in which a nurse talks with a patient with cancer depends on not only her commitment to help and her communication skills but also her knowledge about cancer as an illness, the therapy, and the many ways in which the quality of living can be changed, even when the length of life is limited. Even with all this knowledge, she still must come to grips with her own feelings about pain, death, helplessness, grief, and loss.

Ideally, the patient, the family when appropriate, the physician, and the nurse plan together for care. They may or may not discuss the diagnosis openly with the patient, but there is a general understanding of what he knows and how his part in the treatment has been defined.

When this ideal is not possible, good progress notes by physicians and nurses make possible more meaningful talk with the patient. Lacking notes, the nurse can still learn from the patient what his perception of the situation may be.

Soon after a diagnosis is made, the patient may talk freely of cancer and his treatment. If metastasis is found later, he may no longer be able to call his disease by name.

A simple, open-ended question lets the patient set the pace. When the patient is aware of his diagnosis and the gravity of his situation, he is comforted by talking about his feelings and by the nurse's *listening* and helping him talk. Only when he defines the present situation can he plan the next step. When he does not know his diagnosis or does not wish to discuss it, he will indicate the fact.

Nurses encounter some patients who will not respond to a simple question, who do not wish to talk, or who are unable to do so for some reason. When he is not ready to discuss his condition, a patient may be able to reply to questions about his comfort: "Are you warm enough?" "Do you need more light?" "Do you want a drink?"

A patient who is too sick, too tired, or too depressed to talk may be comforted if the nurse talks quietly to him, explaining what she does, bringing small events of the outside world into the room, keeping him in touch with the present. At times, it is enough for the nurse to be present and to indicate by words, at intervals, that she is there.

Для Improved Service

In recent years, much has been written about the planned use of talking to help patients in pain, patients facing unpleasant treatments, anxious, frightened patients, and terminally ill patients. To carry out care plans requires continuity in contact between nurse and patient and a consistent approach by nurses and physicians. Reports of studies can help nurses increase their knowledge and satisfaction with the care they give. The more a nurse works with patients who have cancer, the more skillful she becomes and the more she appreciates how much the patient brings to each interaction.

Periodic process recording is time consuming, but can help a nurse become aware of what is going on as she talks with patients. These recordings can form the basis for discussion with her co-workers, as they all increase their skills. Also, they can be used to demonstrate progress.

There is much that any nurse can do to insure that even limited contacts are helpful to a patient with cancer. She can give information and instructions simply and clearly. She can get feedback by asking the patient what has been said, to determine that her message did get across. She can listen to what the patient says, attend to his other forms of communication, check her perceptions of his meanings, and let him know that she does, indeed, understand.

To do these things, a nurse comes close to a patient and risks discomfort. At the same time, she learns that when she relieves the patient's loneliness, she herself ceases to work alone. Together, the patient and the nurse can alleviate problems, which neither could manage alone.

Note. From "Talking With Persons Who Have Cancer," by J.K. Craytor, 1969, *American Journal of Nursing, 69*, pp. 744–748. Copyright 1969 by Lippincott Williams & Wilkins. Excerpted with permission.

THE NURSE AND THE CANCER PATIENT: A PROGRAMMED TEXTBOOK (1970)

Preface

Cancer is a major health problem of the modern world. Last year, heart disease, cancer and stroke accounted for seven out of every ten deaths, and together they claimed 1.2 million American lives. If present trends continue, 1 in 4 Americans will have cancer during his life, and cancer will occur in about 2 out of 3 American families.

On the other hand, 33 percent of all persons afflicted with cancer will be alive five years after they are treated. Although the proportions of deaths from cancer rose steadily between 1900 and 1955, it has remained relatively constant since that time due to improved knowledge, understanding, and methods of care, treatment, and detection. Although cancer is a disease of unknown etiology, of almost certain fatal outcome if untreated, and without a specific therapy, experts in the field have confidence that in time the proportion of deaths from cancer can be greatly reduced.

While further progress against the disease depends on discovering the "cause" of cancer, and on specific anticancer treatment methods, less obvious but nevertheless significant obstacles to better progress in the fight against cancer are ignorance and fear. Common unanswered or unasked questions that impede improved results in the fight against cancer include "What is Cancer? Can it be cured? Do cancer patients always die of their disease? How long do they live? What's the use of trying to help? What could I do or say? Is cancer catching?" Erroneous assumptions about the answers to these and other questions are commonly made not only by the general population, patients and their families, but by members of the health care professions as well. The implications of false information or negative attitudes are obvious.

This program is meant to help you find the answers to these questions for yourself. It gives information to enable you to act on your answers, and to help others answer the questions for themselves. It is based on the conviction that your efforts can make a difference. You can play a significant role in seeing that some precancerous changes are avoided or reversed. You can improve the chances for cure by helping patients seek and get early treatment of tumors of limited spread. You can help patients with incurable disease continue to lead a relatively normal and productive life for long periods of time. Even with the rare patient who is suffering a rapid downhill course, your compassionate care and efforts to prevent complications can make the difference between his dying in great pain, with anxiety, or completely disabled, and his ability to face death with dignity and peace of mind.

As part of the health team, you play a role in assessing the physical, emotional, and health teaching needs of the cancer patient and his family. You help to plan his care, carry it out, and evaluate the effectiveness of the care given. This programmed textbook provides you with experiences and problems with patients and other significant persons, which as closely as possible approximate those you would encounter in hospitals, in clinics, and in the community. These people are from every walk of life, present many different problems, and are selected to represent typical situations which vary according to age, sex, personality, type of cancer, stage of disease, treatment methods, and other factors. The case histories are based on actual experiences with patients. The names have been changed to protect the privacy of the individuals involved.

Factual information and general principles required to solve these problems are presented as necessary, although from time to time you may need to draw on your general nursing knowledge. You will learn that the care of the patient with cancer is similar in many ways to the care of any patient, but also it is a challenging area of specialization.

Primarily, we hope that you will find this program interesting. We hope that it will arouse your sense of compassion and strengthen your sense of self-confidence and resolve in fighting the cancer problem. Finally, we hope that it will raise as many new questions as it answers, adding to your motivation to become an increasingly effective member of the health team.

Note. From *The Nurse and the Cancer Patient: A Programmed Textbook* (pp. *v–vi*) by J.K. Craytor and M. Fass, 1970, New York: Lippincott Williams and Wilkins. Copyright 1970 by Lippincott Williams and Wilkins. Reprinted with permission.

TRIBUTES

I entered the junior year of my bachelor's program in nursing at the University of Rochester in 1963. Mrs. Craytor was one of my medical-surgical nursing instructors that year and supervised me in an outpatient clinic experience in the spring of 1964.

By then, Mrs. Craytor had developed the specialized clinical role in cancer nursing that she began exploring in the Medical Center in the late 1950s. She routinely collaborated with physicians in clinical rounds, developing a "team" model of nurse-physician collaboration in the care of patients with cancer. Her experience, based on this model, was the subject of her master's thesis, "An Action Research Project: An Experimental Physician-Nurse Approach to Patient Care." During that year, she began to take more formal responsibility for improving the care of patients with cancer in the medical center. She developed close working relationships with physicians, social workers, and others involved in the care of patients with cancer, instructed undergraduate nursing and medical students and hospital staff in the nursing care of patients with cancer, and participated in community cancer programs. One of her responsibilities during that time included the development of new educational approaches. Working collaboratively with colleagues in the College of Education, she implemented a series of educational research projects designed to develop programmed instruction materials in cancer and cancer care. This work resulted in numerous articles and culminated in the first programmed text in cancer care, *The Nurse and the Cancer Patient: A Programmed Text*.

As an undergraduate student, I was not fully aware of the scope and innovativeness of her work. My experience with these activities was very personal. I was one of the first students to use the programmed instruction materials. The supervised outpatient clinic experience that year was a pivotal point in my career. I had been assigned to care for a young man, an adolescent diabetic, whom I arranged to talk with in the waiting room for several consecutive visits. At Mrs. Craytor's suggestion, I shared my observations and assessments with the patient's physician, Dr. Stan Friedman, each time before he saw the patient. I also sat in on the visit and participated with him and the patient in making a joint plan of care. The relationship I developed with the patient seemed to be helpful; Dr. Friedman and I also worked well together. Unfortunately, the clinic experience was of short duration. Mrs. Craytor suggested and arranged a chance for me to continue my work with the patient and Dr. Friedman in an individualized, extended clinical experience. Dr. Friedman and Mrs. Craytor critiqued a paper I wrote about the nurse-physician collaborative experience in the care of the patient. This was the first of several formative educational experiences that led me to focus the main part of my research career on the interprofessional delivery of health care.

Mrs. Craytor became a lifelong mentor to me after I completed the undergraduate program. During my clinical experiences as a public health nurse for the Monroe County Health Department in Rochester, I provided home care for several challenging patients with cancer. When I

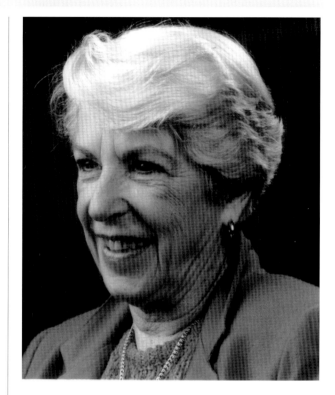

ABOVE
Josephine Craytor

JOSEPHINE K. CRAYTOR

needed advice, I called Mrs. Craytor. Some of these experiences stand out in my mind as crucial learning experiences even almost 35 years later.

The challenges I encountered in public health nursing led me to recognize a need for more education. I did not complete a master's degree in a clinical specialty. (These programs were extremely new and rare when I returned to graduate school in 1967.) I was encouraged to apply for a Federal Special Nurse Research Fellowship to support graduate work in a discipline allied to nursing. Based on interest and my community health nursing experience, I decided to study sociology, first at the University of Rochester and then at the State University of New York at Buffalo, where I focused on small-group theory and research. Mrs. Craytor's persistence in keeping me connected to nursing throughout my graduate training kept me from straying from nursing. She was teaching a graduate seminar in the small medical-surgical nursing master's program at the University of Rochester. Periodically, she called me and invited me to come and talk to her students about what I was studying and its relevance to nursing.

Eventually, I accepted a position at the School of Nursing at the University of Rochester. Mrs. Craytor became my colleague. She fostered my career through informal support and formal connections. She was a sponsor for my application to the American Academy of Nursing in 1977. In the early 1980s, when she completed her term on the National Cancer Institute Clinical Cancer Education Review Committee, she recommended me as her replacement. She supported my interest in applying my small-group skills gained in graduate school to research and clinical facilitation of patients with cancer and family support groups.

Mrs. Craytor is a master clinical teacher and mentor who recognized how to foster students' development and interest in cancer nursing care, in academic life and in life in general. She and Russ have been a model for how to live life to the fullest. After retirement, Mrs. Craytor has continued to be active in the care of patients, first as a Friend of Strong (Memorial Hospital) volunteer and now through the School of Nursing at Rochester, working to foster wellness and healthcare programs in her retirement community. She has continued to be a key source of professional advice and counsel to me throughout the years, even now as I begin to contemplate my own retirement. Besides important conversation, she and Russ offer their cottage to me as a retreat from my hectic schedule and as a place for concentrated work. She says it is the place where she always worked best.

Madeline H. Schmitt, RN, PhD, FAAN

*Professor of Nursing, Independence Chair in Nursing,
and Interprofessional Education and Coordinator
Doctoral Program
University of Rochester, NY*

I first met Jo Craytor in 1975 when I was finishing the RN-BS program at the University of Rochester. Because I was planning to enter the master's degree Medical-Surgical Nursing program in the fall and had some interest in cancer nursing, Jo encouraged me to apply for a summer Cancer Nursing Fellowship sponsored by the United Cancer Council, Inc. (now Cancer Action, Inc.). Jo was instrumental in developing this fellowship for the purpose of giving students an opportunity to explore the cancer-nursing role and to cultivate interest specializing in advanced-cancer nursing. For me, this was the beginning of three very rich years of learning about cancer nursing from Jo, the cancer clinical nurse specialist (CNS) role, commitment to generating and disseminating cancer nursing knowledge, professional networking with other cancer nurses and healthcare providers, and mentoring. In all of these areas, Jo set an excellent example, sharing both her successes and struggles to overcome difficulties.

One of Jo's strengths was her ability to integrate teaching and mentoring in a way that taught the substantive content, fostered active learning, promoted student self-esteem and independence, and modeled the professional role she expected of us. For example, while I was learning about cancer nursing and the CNS role in the master's program, staff nurses needed to learn more about the care of patients with cancer undergoing state-of-the-art therapy. Consequently, as students, we had many opportunities grounded in the "real world" to learn to be educators, change agents, and consultants as well as direct-care providers. During this time, I was Jo's research assistant. She actively involved me in all phases of the research process, including joint authorship of two articles written about the study.

After graduation, I worked under Jo as a cancer CNS. During this time, she supported my growth as an advanced clinician as well as fostered my commitment to the specialty of oncology nursing. She encouraged our group of four CNSs to submit abstracts, present, and attend the fledgling Oncology Nursing Society (ONS). She also encouraged our active involvement on committees in ONS as well as in other cancer organizations, such as the American Association of Cancer Education (AACE). I remember vividly her networking and mentoring when attending my first AACE meeting with her in New Orleans. I was in awe when she introduced me to people like Virginia Barckley and Louise Lunceford and encouraged me to participate in the conversation by telling them a little about something I was doing. My awe quickly was overcome, however, when I noted the camaraderie these oncology nurses shared and their warm welcome of newcomers to cancer nursing.

Of the many teachers I have had, Jo has had the greatest influence on the professional that I am today. I try to follow her example in many aspects of my work, especially in teaching and mentoring students. Critical behaviors I learned from Jo that have influenced me the most are to ground my teaching in the real world, mentor students in a collegial manner, and collaborate with local and national colleagues to improve cancer care through the generation and dissemination of new knowledge. Jo is a first-class teacher, mentor, and cancer nursing professional who pioneered the advanced practice oncology-nursing role. It is a privilege to have been her student.

Jean K. Brown, RN, PhD
Associate Professor
State University of New York
Buffalo, NY

Professional papers and effects of Josephine Craytor are located in the archives of the Medical Library at the University of Rochester, NY, and in the archives at the National Office of the Oncology Nursing Society in Pittsburgh, PA.

FLORENCE SCHORSKE WALD, RN, BA, MN, MS
Leader in Research and Development of the Hospice Movement in the United States

"What people need most when they are dying is relief from distressing symptoms of their disease, the security of a caring environment, sustained expert care, and the assurance they and their families won't be abandoned."

— *Florence Schorske Wald*

FLORENCE SCHORSKE WALD

BIOGRAPHICAL INFORMATION

BIRTH

Florence Schorske was born at home in Bronx, NY, on April 19, 1917.

PARENTS

Florence Schorske's family had strong Germanic values that shaped her life and heavily influenced her professional accomplishments. Florence was the second child of Theodore and Gertrude (Goldschmidt) Schorske. Her only sibling, Carl, was born two years before Florence. Her parents both were born in New York City; Theodore was German Catholic, and Gertrude was Jewish. They knew the value of education, and although formal education was unaffordable, they immersed themselves in all that the city had to offer, becoming versed in art, music, theatre, history, politics, and literature. Theodore became a banker and also gave generously of his time in support of new immigrants to the United States. He volunteered in the city's neighborhoods to help immigrants acclimate to life in the United States. Gertrude's "second home" was the Brooklyn Public Library.

FAMILY

The Schorske family traveled a great deal, including trips to Europe, on which the children were included. Carl and Florence enjoyed the same exposure to all of New York's great cultural attractions that their parents did. To further enhance the children's education, the family left the Bronx, moving to Scarsdale, NY, where the school system had a reputation for excellence.

Carl was enrolled at Columbia University studying history when Florence graduated from high school. At this point, her father's Germanic values, as Florence described them, became an obstacle to her. Money was not the issue. Theodore did not believe that formal education beyond high school was necessary for girls, and he did not want to send Florence to college. Carl believed otherwise and joined their mother in "ganging up" on Theodore to convince him to allow Florence to attend college.

Fortunately, their efforts were successful, and Florence enrolled at Mt. Holyoke College in Massachusetts to study physiology and sociology. Carl went on to a very distinguished academic career at Princeton University and is now Professor Emeritus at Princeton. Florence and Carl remained very close throughout their lives.

CAREER PATH

Florence knew when she entered college that she wanted to be a nurse. Influenced by her "big sister" at Mt. Holyoke who had attended Yale, Florence enrolled in Yale's master's program in nursing after graduating from Mt. Holyoke in 1938 with a bachelor of art degree. Another factor in Florence's decision to attend Yale was the work accomplished by Annie Goodrich, founder of the Yale nursing program, who had consulted at Mt. Holyoke and helped to develop the basic science classes there in physiology, zoology, and chemistry.

At the time, the nursing program at Yale was three years in length, included extensive clinical experience, and led to a master's degree in nursing. Florence still believes that without an intensely clinical program at the master's-degree level, today's baccalaureate-prepared nursing students are at a distinct disadvantage when enrolled in master's-degree study. She has observed that the individual who first acquires basic nursing training followed by a bachelor's degree in nursing or related field is far better prepared clinically than those who only graduate from a bachelor's program. She noted that the latter group is at a disadvantage in today's master's programs because of the minimal clinical experience at both levels.

VISITING NURSE SERVICE

Following graduation from the Yale School of Nursing in 1941, Florence wanted to join the war effort with a medical unit from Yale. However, her parents, who were pacifists, would not agree with this, and, so instead, Florence went to work in public health with the Henry Street Visiting Nurse Service in New York City. Nursing in this setting was not as she had anticipated it to be, as she saw technology and administration dominating nursing practice. After 18 months, she left to work for the Army Signal Corp in a research project at Columbia University College of Physicians and Surgeons. The research involved the study of life at extreme temperatures, with soldiers in officer's training serving as the research subjects. One of these soldiers was Henry Wald. In Florence's words, "We enjoyed a nice relationship." However, when Henry proposed, Florence turned him down, knowing that she was still searching for her direction in life and was not ready for marriage. Florence continued with her work in research, focusing next on development of techniques for corneal transplants. The war in Europe escalated, and at the time of the Battle of the Bulge, Florence could no longer ignore her desire to be a part of the war effort. She signed on as an Army nurse and was assigned to West Point Military Academy, where she worked on an obstetrical ward for the next year.

Florence's interest turned to psychiatry, and when Yale opened a master's degree program in psychiatry, she enrolled. Although some clinical experience was included, Florence felt that the program was not focused. She became a teaching assistant to Hildegard Peplau at Rutgers University and happily found the first nursing theory that she could truly embrace, Peplau's theory of interpersonal relationships.

The strength of their relationship is revealed in the following passage from a publication that Carl Schorske dedicated to his sister, Florence.

Companion through life,

ever-courageous

ever-supportive

ever-comprehending

sister beloved,

How great to walk on

separate paths yet

always together

in heart and mind!

SCHORSKE, C. (1998). *THINKING WITH HISTORY: EXPLORATIONS IN THE PASSAGE TO MODERNISM.* PRINCETON, NJ: PRINCETON UNIVERSITY PRESS.

FLORENCE SCHORSKE WALD

BELOW
Florence and Henry Wald

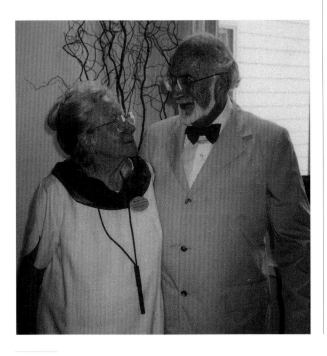

The year was 1956, and in Florence's words, "Yale was having trouble." President A. Whitney Griswold did not believe that training practitioners (i.e., engineers, teachers, nurses) suited the image of an academic institution. Therefore, he had closed the schools of education and nursing. Florence joined the alumni group in launching a vigorous protest, and President Griswold rescinded his decision. He also challenged the nursing faculty to design a new master's degree program in nursing. Dean Elizabeth Bixler asked Florence to return to Yale to help redesign the psychiatric nursing component with Marion Russell, the lead instructor. Marion resigned shortly thereafter, and Florence became lead instructor. Sensing a degree of inertia in the total program redesign, Florence and other faculty members assembled at the home of Ernestine Weidenbach (of the midwifery faculty) in Bethlehem, CT. The result was a new master's in nursing program known as "The Bethlehem Document."

Elizabeth Bixler left Yale, and Florence was named acting dean. She was faced with the challenge of getting the redesigned nursing program up and running. Virginia Henderson arrived at Yale and promoted her strong belief in researching nursing problems, not nurses. Florence, whose office adjoined Virginia's, found her to be a great friend, supportive colleague, and advisor. Robert Leonard, a Yale sociologist, also was very important to Florence at that time because he helped nursing students to design their research using small groups for comparative studies.

YALE SCHOOL OF NURSING

In 1959, Florence was named Dean of the Yale School of Nursing. The announcement of this appointment, along with her picture, appeared in the *New York Times*. Henry Wald happened to notice the picture as he glanced at another person's newspaper. He lost no time in contacting Florence. Henry was now a very successful engineering consultant and owned a firm that specialized in illumination of public buildings. He had married and was the father of two children, whom he had been raising alone after the tragic death of his wife in a car accident. This time, when Henry proposed marriage, Florence said yes. At the age of 41, Florence married Henry and became the mother to 6-year-old Shari and 8-year-old Joel. Florence said that she always thinks of the words to the hymn "Amazing Grace" when she reflects on the circumstances of her marriage to her beloved husband, Henry: "I once was lost, but now am found."

Joel Wald, his wife, and two children live in New York where he is a business consultant who helps companies to develop and express new ideas. Shari lives in Nova Scotia with her husband and their three children. Shari, a registered nurse, practices Tibetan Buddhism and provides spiritual care in the hospital system with an interfaith consultation group.

As Dean of the Yale School of Nursing during the 1960s, Florence observed with keen interest the differences in students admitted to Yale's master's degree program based upon their undergraduate preparation. She believed in the need for extensive clinical experience "for one to really begin to see what nursing questions are. What are the nursing acts that help patients? And, why do they help?" Florence was concerned that in most nursing programs, "the theoretical and conceptual . . . the lengthy discussion of theories of nursing, doesn't really touch on what the basic problems are." She is proud of the fact that during her years at Yale, the nursing program was very patient and family oriented. In their intensive, frequent, and close contact with patients and families, nursing students observed the doctor-patient relationship, noting that difficulties occurred, particularly in communication. Patients were asking nurses and students questions about their illness and what lay ahead for them, and doctors would not permit nurses to answer. "Doctors and nurses moved in parallel tracks rather than collaboratively in teams. The dissatisfactions with each other were usually unspoken" (Wald, 1997).

During the 1960s, Florence also observed the long-needed coalescence of the social sciences, a vital force in what would later become the hospice movement. Professionals in sociology, psychology, nursing, political science, anthropology, and other disciplines worked together and examined their roles in influencing health and the course of illness. Dr. Max Pepper (Yale School of Public Health and Department of Sociology), along with his wife, Anita (a social worker), were leaders in the work to establish community mental health centers during the move to deinstitutionalize the mentally ill.

A pivotal event in 1963 ultimately changed Florence's direction and led to her well-known work with the hospice movement. Virginia Henderson invited Florence to attend a presentation by Cicely Saunders, leader of the hospice movement in the United Kingdom, who was delivering the program to Yale medical school students. Florence was unable to attend, but immediately following the speech, Virginia "was ecstatic" and regaled Florence with the significance of the message that Saunders had delivered, noting that the medical students "had even stood up, clapped, and cheered!" Florence arranged to have Saunders repeat her presentation the following day for a hastily assembled audience from the hospital, nursing school, and school of social work. Florence stated, "After meeting and hearing Cicely Saunders, I was hooked."

Many individuals were beginning to ask the question, "How are we handling death and dying?" Elizabeth Kübler-Ross became widely known for her perception of the human response to imminent death as a series of stages. Jeanne Quint Benoliel published the results of her research on the impact of mastectomy, identifying concerns about shortened life and slow, painful death as being foremost in women's minds. "Spiritual support in illness that had disappeared in the age of

FLORENCE SCHORSKE WALD

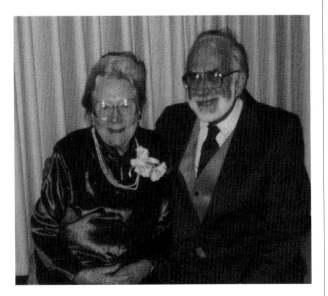

ABOVE
Florence and Henry Wald

enlightenment in the 18th and 19th centuries returned with the active role that churches and divinity schools played in the community in the early 1960s. Departments of religious ministries were established in hospitals, and divinity students learned to give spiritual support (to the hospitalized)" (Wald, 1997).

In 1965, enroute to Europe on the SS Rotterdam with her husband and children, Florence "decided mid-ocean, to change focus and go back to clinical nursing." She recognized that being part of a two-income family with a very supportive husband made the decision both easier and possible. In 1968, Florence resigned as dean and began the research that led to her identification of the great need for hospice care. On a subsequent family trip to Europe, Florence worked for three weeks at St. Christopher's Hospice in London while Henry and the children were sightseeing.

Florence served as principal investigator for the following two studies (unpublished), which provided the evidence base upon which she and her colleagues moved forward to establish hospice services in Connecticut.

- A Nurse's Study of Care for Dying Patients, USPHS Grant NU 00352, Principal Investigator, 10/1/69–9/30/71.
- An Interdisciplinary Study of Care for Dying Patients and Their Families, ANF Grant No. 2-70-032, Principal Investigator, 2/1/70–1/31/71

Patients for the studies were identified through the office of Dr. Ira Goldenberg, Professor of Surgery at Yale. Goldenberg, who treated many women with breast cancer, was well known among his medical and nursing colleagues for his dedication to caring for his patients, even when treatment and surgery had failed to bring about cure. Florence provided nursing care to the terminally ill in any setting (e.g., home, hospital, nursing home) for any patient who agreed to allow her to take notes as a participant observer. She was joined by Katherine Klause for a portion of the study, in which a total of 22 patients were cared for and observed during the two-year research period. Katherine, a private duty nurse, brought her highly developed clinical skills to this team effort, complementing Florence's expert interpersonal skills. Florence described a number of events and individual contributions in addition to these two studies that formed the basis for the hospice movement in Connecticut.

During this period, a group of individuals had been meeting on a regular basis to share their common interest in the needs of the terminally ill. In addition to Florence and her husband, the group included Katherine Klause, Dr. Goldenberg, Dr. Morris Wessel (pediatrician), Rev. Edward Dobihal (Methodist minister), Father Robert Canney (Roman Catholic priest), and Rev. Frederick Auman (Lutheran minister). Each contributed to the development and eventual establishment of the Hospice for the Greater New Haven Region, which later became known as The Connecticut

Hospice, Inc. in Branford, CT. This dedicated group of individuals, with a common interest in improving care for the dying, constituted the Founding Board of Directors.

Henry Wald's growing involvement in hospice led him to close his engineering consultant practice in 1970 and enroll in the School of Architecture at Columbia University, majoring in health facilities planning. He later would conduct the feasibility study for the siting and construction of the Branford hospice facility.

Wessel published an article (about the need for a new approach to the care of the terminally ill) in the Yale alumni magazine, in which he included a quotation from Maimonides (rabbi, physician, Jewish philosopher): "... to cure sometimes, to comfort, always ..." Members of the Van Ameringen Foundation responded to that article with an offer of financial support for the hospice movement, as well as referral to other potential donors. Saunders returned to Yale as a visiting faculty member and helped various groups to coalesce. The Yale School of Nursing provided office space for the hospice planning work.

In 1974, the first patients were admitted to the Hospice Home Care program, which operated out of space in the nursing school, then in the New Haven Church of the Redeemer, and later at Albertus Magnus College—all provided rent-free. Planning for an inpatient facility continued as many community volunteers joined committees of the Board along with members of the Hospice Home Care staff to work on various aspects such as building and site development, licensing, patient care, staff selection, spirituality, research, professional and community collaboration, and fund-raising. Planning was heavily influenced by an unstable political climate and sweeping changes in health care throughout the country. In addition to the process of obtaining a Certificate of Need (CON), there was uncertainty about the type of licensure required for this new and unique healthcare facility. The Board agreed to bring in a politically astute and seasoned consultant to move the licensing and CON process along. The consultant was successful, and when his task was accomplished, he proposed that an administrator should be hired immediately to manage and direct all aspects of the continued planning, construction, and facilities management. Florence adamantly disagreed with his recommendation. The Board had planned to hire an administrator once the hospice facility was opened, but that individual would be carrying out the work as

BELOW
Florence and Henry Wald

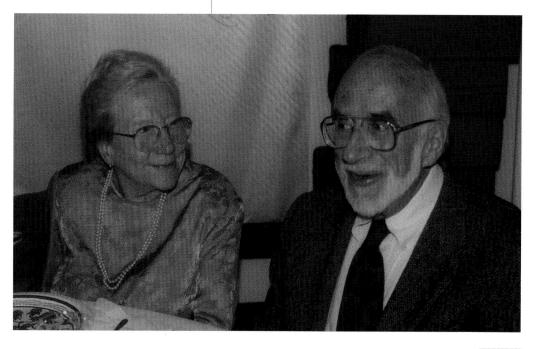

directed by the Board. Florence held fast to her belief that the hospice could be run democratically, with committee and community group participation, as it had throughout the planning and development. The Board, however, agreed with the consultant's recommendation and immediately voted to hire him to serve as the new administrator.

Henry and Florence left for a vacation in England, and, upon their return, the administrator met with Florence to review all that had taken place in her absence. He carefully described all that had been accomplished under his direction and concluded by telling her that because of their differences in operational philosophy, either she would need to resign from the Board, or he would leave. When the Board put their support behind the administrator, Florence bowed out in 1975.

As painful and difficult as her separation was from the Hospice for the Greater New Haven Region, Florence was able to reconcile these events with the help and support of Henry and her family. She realized that she was "out of sync" with the administrator's political style as well as with his top-down approach to management. In addition, after lengthy discussion with Seymour Sarason, a Yale colleague and consulting psychologist, Florence understood that what was happening in her relationship with the Board and staff was part of the "phenomenon of growth" that occurs when societies create new organizations. "Blending the skills of many professions in a responsibly sharing team, most members of which are accustomed to a traditional hierarchy, requires a different and an additional social adjustment" (Wald, Foster, & Wald, 1980). Using the analogy of the theatre, Sarason likened Florence's position to one in which the author/playwright (Florence) tries to influence the play's director (the hospice administrator) and the actors (staff and committees) in the production and staging of the play. It is seldom successful.

The Branford hospice facility opened in 1980. Henry Wald, Virginia Henderson, and others on the Building and Site Committee selected the architectural firm for this pioneering venture, based upon the firm's interest in new ideas and willingness to incorporate the committee's ideas. The architects visited St. Christopher's Hospice in London and St. Luke's in Sheffield, England, in addition to reviewing extensive minutes from the Hospice Board and committee meetings. The Connecticut Hospice, Inc. (as it was named in 1999) stands in peaceful, wooded surroundings in Branford, CT, the first inpatient hospice in the United States. In addition to the inpatient facility, which accommodates 52 patients, a homecare program also flourishes.

BELOW
Florence and Henry Wald

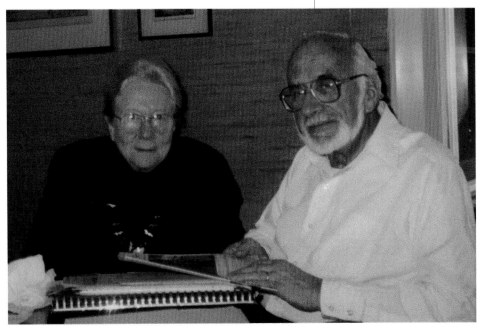

Florence was asked to return as a volunteer, which she did willingly, and she worked with the interdisciplinary staff from 1980–1983, looking at the issues surrounding coma and delirium in patients. Florence also continued active involvement with an international group that had been meeting regularly to discuss death and dying. She was an eloquent spokesperson for the hospice concept, and a much-sought-after speaker. This group, The International Work Group (IWG) on Death, Dying, and Bereavement was founded in 1974 and continues to meet every 18 months. Florence and Henry were among the 50 founding members of this dedicated group. Florence chaired the Spiritual Care Workgroup that developed the Assumptions and Principles of Spiritual Care (Corless et al., 1990). This guide for healthcare providers addresses the spiritual dimensions of a person's life and presents the principles upon which support and respect for spirituality can and must be incorporated into care of the dying.

Florence had difficulty with her own lack of what she could identify as a religious base. Her father (born of Catholic and Lutheran parents) was an avowed atheist, who led many family dinner table discussions on the subject of religion. He felt that organized religion and religious leaders made it very difficult for people to express individuality in their lives when adhering to any specific doctrine. Florence's mother was Jewish; and as a result of these childhood influences, Florence grew up with a knowledge base in comparative religion but with no spiritual direction of her own. This became a major personal issue as she began her work with the hospice movement, especially under the tutelage of Cicely Saunders. Saunders was steeped in the Anglican faith, and St. Christopher's Hospice was considered ecumenical Christian. Religious faith was an essential component of St. Christopher's concept of hospice care. During the 1980s, a number of people and events came together and enabled Florence to resolve this long-held personal dilemma.

Florence took note of the work of the psychologist Samuel Klagsbrun, who was very interested in hospice and supported Saunders' belief in the necessity for a religious foundation for hospice care. He maintained that hospice caregivers need to understand what their own spiritual resources are to provide comprehensive care to patients. Another influence arose even closer to home for Florence when she delved into understanding her daughter, Shari's, interest in Tibetan Buddhism. Florence was challenged to examine her own question of "Where do I stand on religion and faith?" These thoughts and questions were brought back to the Spiritual Care Workgroup of the IWG on Death, Dying, and Bereavement to explore the common elements of both religious and secular spirituality. From this fruitful sharing of so many religious and lay representatives, there emerged for Florence "a breakthrough . . . a realization and understanding that my own spiritual basis was rooted in the arts."

Although Florence separated from the Connecticut Hospice organization a number of years ago, her influence, expertise, and interest in and commitment to the care of the dying has not

---

Florence's work and dedication has not gone unnoticed. She has been the recipient of many honors and honorary degrees.

Doctor of Law, 1967
University of Bridgeport School of Nursing

Distinguished Woman of Connecticut Award, 1976
Governor of Connecticut

Doctor of Humane Letters, 1978
Mt. Holyoke College

Fellow, 1979
American Academy of Nursing

First Recipient of the Florence S. Wald Award for Contribution to Nursing Practice, 1980
Connecticut Nurses' Association

Founders Award, 1987
National Hospice Organization

Contribution to Hospice Award, 1990
National Association of Home Care

Honorary Degree of Medical Sciences, 1995
Yale University

Induction
American Nurses Association Hall of Fame, 1996

The National Women's Hall of Fame, 1998

The Connecticut Women's Hall of Fame, 1999

FLORENCE SCHORSKE WALD

ended. Inspired by the work of a prisoner, Fleet Maull (who has since been pardoned), Florence has become involved in hospice activities within prison walls, which Maull helped to organize. A student of Tibetan Buddhism, Maull had started ministering to the needs of his fellow prisoners who were dying. He and other prisoners essentially became hospice volunteers within the prison walls. Word of his work spread, and, in 1989, the National Prison Hospice Association was formed. In 1996, Florence and two associates, Diane Robbins (a nursing student at that time) and Nealy Zimmermann (an accountant and member of the Tibetan Buddhist community), conducted a feasibility study, visiting all of Connecticut's state prisons. They reviewed the needs of dying inmates and explored ways of connecting community resources with the prisoners' hospice needs. Florence believes that "the most important thing about the prison hospice movement is that we are reaching a completely different sector of society, one that we are constantly putting aside and forgetting about, just as we did for psychiatric patients for so many years."

SUMMARY

Florence Wald is truly a nursing pioneer in her tireless efforts to bring hospice care into reality in the United States. Her deep sense of humanity, her courageous stand and willingness to take risks, and her inspired insight into the needs of the dying are embodied in the founding of the first U.S. hospice program in Connecticut. Her name remains synonymous with hospice care. Florence resides in her Connecticut home following the death of her husband in December 2000.

REFERENCES

Corless, I., Wald, F.S., Autton, N., Bailey, S., Cosh, R., Cockburn, M., Head, D., DeVeber, B., DeVeber, I., Ley, C., Mauritzen, J., Nichols, J., O'Connor, P., & Saito, T. (1990). Assumptions and principles of spiritual care. *Death Studies, 14*, 75–81.

Duff, R.S., & Hollingshead, A.B. (1968). *Sickness and society*. New York: Harper and Row.

Wald, F.S. (1997). Hospice's path to the future. In S. Strack (Ed.), *Death and the quest for meaning. Essays in honor of Herman Feifel* (pp. 57–77). Northvale, NJ: Jason Aronson Inc.

Wald, F.S., Foster, Z., & Wald, H.J. (1980). The hospice movement as a health care reform. *Nursing Outlook, 28*, 173–178.

Wald, Florence, interview by Laura Hilderley, June 1999.

SELECTED WRITING
HOSPICE'S PATH TO THE FUTURE (1997)

Care for the terminally ill is one part of the health care system in the United States that has been transformed, beginning in the 1960's. It came into being as health care providers witnessed the neglect and suffering of those patients who do not improve with intensive scientific medical therapy. Hospice care, also called palliative care, is one of several patient-centered approaches that depends on more than medical science, visualizes the whole person, the family, social conditions, and the soul as well as the body in its scope to understand health and disease.

While medical care in the twentieth century has been dominated by basic science, medical science, and technology, the social sciences, ethics, the nature of man, and the nature of suffering are emerging as key issues in a counterculture.

Looking back on health policy in the twentieth century, dominant values were in balance with opposing values of a counterculture.

Awakening health professionals and the public to alternative ways of caring for terminally ill patients and families happened suddenly and spread widely beginning in the 1960's. St. Christopher's Hospice in England opened in 1967; the first services for the terminally ill did not begin in the United States until 1974. However, groundwork was laid in the decade of the 1960's when penetrating questions and answers called for change in many institutions—government, religion, education and medicine.

In academia, there was a surge of interest following World War II in death and dying that brought the field of thanatology into being.

Health professionals became aware of the tremendous cost and suffering accompanying catastrophic and life-threatening illnesses as they faced the rise of an aging population. In an age when technology dominated mainstream medical practice there was also a call for care that recognized the whole patient, whose suffering was broader than physical suffering and whose family suffered, too. How did a call for change arise, challenge traditional medicine, and create an alternative approach?

Although it was technology that dominated the medical world after World War II and attracted the majority of caregivers, nevertheless there was a significant minority whose focus was on the whole person, in whom psyche and soma interact, whose health affects and is affected by family, whose coping skills were determined by lifestyle and one's place in community. There was a counter-culture that thought of the patient and family first and then adapting medical intervention to it.

While hospitals' rules, regulations, schedules, and environment were composed to make the work of doctors and nurses run smoothly, after World War II dissident caregivers called for space and services to include family and put patients first.

From the changing relationship of patients and caregivers, the issue of rights of patients arose. Physicians in a position of power gave much thought to what and who influenced the choice of treatment . . . Putting medical ethics into practice proved daunting. . .

Ethics committees were formed in hospitals with physicians, nurses, ethicists and lawyers participating to consider the options in a particular case. What are the treatment alternatives? What does the patient know and want? What impact will it have on the patient/family quality of life? These discussions gave a picture of the whole person in the context of his relationship with family and other important people in his/her life.

The medical profession took a long time to integrate the relationship of soma and psyche . . .

Nursing took the body and soul or mind seriously, although it was a difficult relationship to trace in scientific inquiry.

. . . Doctors, lawyers, nurses, ethicists studied and revamped the roles of patients and caregivers in terms of moral responsibility and patient rights. Patients became partners in being and getting informed and deciding the course of action.

The effect of illness on the whole family became a significant issue in planning care. A broader view of healing and the planning of spiritual support brought other disciplines into the caregiving team. Medical science and medical models of care are no longer the only perspective. The patient has become the whole person in sickness or good health. The physician is a member of an interdisciplinary team.

Changing Care of the Terminally Ill

. . . In hospitals in the 1960's, traditional medical and surgical care for adults prevailed, curative treatment was pursued even when the hoped for cure was not achieved, and the patient's suffering continued. The patient who wanted to cease treatment had to accept discharge from the hospital. It was difficult to change course, even in shifting from one form of therapy to another, such as surgery, radiation and/or chemotherapy for patients with cancer. Seeking a second opinion took courage on the part of a patient, and doctors did not feel obligated to fully explain what medical problem they found, what options there were to correct it, or to engage the patient and family in deciding what to do . . .

Nurses and doctors became increasingly uncomfortable in seeing patients exhausted, depleted, in pain, and frightened.

After St. Christopher's Hospice in London opened its doors in 1967, a few professionals from the United States and Canada gathered work experience there. Professional practitioners and academicians of various disciplines met in conference.

Meanwhile, the public became so enthused about the concepts of palliative and holistic care that new ventures began service and accepted volunteers.

The broader concept of suffering of the dying patient/family infiltrated the medical model. Strategies borrowed from the best of traditional modern medicine, as Saunders emphasized from the beginning, blended with other ways of healing and reducing stress. However, Saunders's position was to maintain and sustain a firm footing in established medicine, and established religion.

In the United States nurses were attracted to and promoted hospice care sooner and more enthusiastically than doctors. Nurses had developed their role as being perceptive of patients' wants and skilled in helping them to express it. Their focus was on the human being with an illness.

The balance between traditional and holistic practitioners in each palliative care/hospice institution shapes the therapeutic thrust. The ability and willingness of doctors and nurses to learn from one another and negotiate, determine how much the process moves forward.

Hope for the Future

If one reviews the [healthcare] problems solved and the emerging new solutions of the twentieth century, health professionals can reshape and restructure approaches based on knowing what works and what doesn't. This is a substantive but difficult revolution.

The medical model would still engage in diagnoses, complex treatments and scientific inquiry with its own space, order, and ethos. Its domain would be smaller, but designed for an ever changing technology. The health support system would have its base in the community, helping patients cope with their own and family illness and keeping well. A bridge between these two is essential to its function: people caring for themselves and for each other to sustain health through the life cycle.

Interim Response to a Changed Health System

It is uncertain what managed care will be like in the year 2000. Some hospices have responded by becoming part of a health care system, not always by choice, but because of coercion and competition by the larger system Others have fortified themselves by merging with other hospices, some resulting in hospice chains or becoming mega-hospices. . .

The hospice movement still has weaknesses. Its wildfire spread fanned by an eager public and zealous founders bypassed careful study of need and existing resources. Not every state requires certificates of need, and those that do have different stipulations.

Organizational forms vary. There are free-standing hospices, palliative care units in hospitals, home care agencies, skilled nursing facilities, hospice teams serving dying nursing home clients, AIDS hospices, residences and services to the homeless in the community, and hospice day care. Interagency relations have taken a variety of forms.

The patients admitted initially were primarily cancer patients. Now there are patients with other diagnoses. Patients with AIDS have an extended trajectory and uneven course. A patient whose crises are severe may unexpectedly go into remission.

Home care in theory makes sense, but for the patient who lives alone or whose helpmate is at work, it is inadequate.

While [hospice] revenues come from multiple sources—government, private insurance, patient, private foundations, contributions, community fund raising, and corporations—deficits and operational costs are a common problem. How many not-for-profit hospices are able to put aside capital funds to guarantee the institutions' security and independence?

Given the knowledge now available about the nature of suffering and holistic care, will government and the society it serves recognize and choose basic health care for all as a right? Can our society strike an equitable balance in its democratic and capitalist values?

Note. From "Hospice's Path to the Future" (pp. 57–77) by F.S. Wald in S. Strack (Ed.), *Death and the Quest for Meaning. Essays in Honor of Herman Feifel,* 1997, Northvale, NJ: Jason Aronson, Inc. Copyright 1997 by Jason Aronson, Inc. Excerpted with permission.

TRIBUTES

Florence Wald, upon her retirement as dean of the Yale University School of Nursing, decided to concentrate her energy and efforts on the improvement of the care of terminally ill patients in this country. She had been particularly concerned with this aspect of health care since 1963, when Cicely Saunders visited Yale and described the movement in London which resulted in the planning and building of St. Christopher's Hospice for the care of patients who were terminally ill and their families.

In 1968, Florence spent three weeks visiting St. Christopher's Hospice. She returned to New Haven determined to create a comparable service in our community. Her first step was to organize an interdisciplinary group of physicians, nurses, clergy, and others to consider various aspects of the care of the terminally ill and their families. I was pleased when Florence invited me to participate in this group.

Dr. Goldenberg, Professor of Surgery at Yale Medical School, well known for his interest in following terminally ill patients to the end of their lives, invited Florence to join him in his daily hospital rounds to observe the care of these patients.

Members of the interdisciplinary study group possessed a reverence for human life and a determination to improve care of the terminally ill and their families. Florence's discussions of her visit in London and her experiences attending the local hospital rounds led the group to support the development of a hospice program in our community. The Hospice for the Greater New Haven Region was formed, which initiated a homecare program in 1974. This provided nursing services and medical consultations to patients and their families at home.

When it became too difficult to care for patients at home, hospitals in our community only offered limited supportive care. I remember meeting with the chief of staff of a local hospital 30 years ago, during which he commented, "We certainly need a hospice when our job is done."

Florence's determination and skilled guidance led the interdisciplinary planning group to plan and construct a building for inpatient services. The Hospice for the Greater New Haven Region in Branford opened in 1980. This 52-bed center was the first building in the United States to be planned and built specifically for serving patients who were terminally ill and their families. As patients, family members, physicians, nurses, or visitors enter the building, overwhelming warmth and peacefulness are felt that reflect the values that Florence communicated in her leadership of the discussions with the interdisciplinary study group. She continues to offer this important leadership by working with the International Work Group on Death, Dying and Bereavement, which is dedicated to offering the collegial support services of physicians, nurses, social workers, and

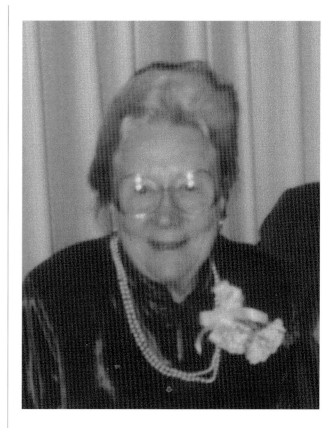

ABOVE
Florence Wald

155

other colleagues to those wishing to provide appropriate services for terminally ill patients and their families at this difficult moment and during bereavement.

Morris A. Wessel, MD

Clinical Professor of Pediatrics
Yale University School of Medicine
New Haven, CT

What strikes me most about Florence is the way people immediately respond to her through actions and words. People want to approach her and talk about their experience and desires. This was made clear to me one day when she and I went to the women's prison in Connecticut on one of our many visits to prisons throughout the state. On this particular visit, we were going to talk with students of a nurse's aide training program, an inmate who had been diagnosed with cancer, and the nurses who worked on the medical unit in the prison. As Florence and I walked into the medical unit, the people working on the unit seemed to flock to her direction without having been summoned.

This type of response happened frequently as people were drawn to her. I am not sure why this happens. Maybe it is because she looks people in the eyes and approaches them without fear, or perhaps it is because of her kind, gentle manner. On that day, the inmates in the aide training program answered our questions with openness and sincerity. The healthcare providers were very interested in the possibility of hospice in the corrections system.

The woman who had been diagnosed with cancer talked with Florence as if they had been buddies for a long time. Even though we were in a circle of people, she maintained eye contact with Florence more than anyone. At the end of our conversation, she reached out to hug Florence and thanked her profusely for her concern.

I have learned a lot from Florence as a nursing student and person. I have learned about the history of nursing, women, nursing school, and life. I am honored to have had the opportunity to work with her, and I am even more honored to be her friend. Ultimately, she confirms the notion that it is possible and imperative that all humans are respected in the process of their life as well as death. This universal respect seems to be a key element to her successful inner and outer life.

Diane Robbins, RN, MSN

Nurse Practitioner
Department of Public Health
HIV Prevention Section
San Francisco, CA

Professional papers and effects of Florence Schorske Wald are located in the Yale University Bioethics Archives in New Haven, CT.

JEANNE QUINT BENOLIEL, RN, DNSc, FAAN
Leader in Cancer Nursing Research and Education

"To have cancer in our society was to bear a stigma. That is, the person with cancer had an undesired attribute which often led to isolation from others in the environment."

— *Jeanne Quint Benoliel*

JEANNE QUINT BENOLIEL

SIGNIFICANT CAREER CONTRIBUTIONS

- Developed the role of a nurse scientist at a time when nurses either took care of patients or taught nursing but never were thought of as researchers

- Investigated the landmark "mastectomy study" funded by the National Institute of Mental Health in 1961. This study examined the adjustment process of women during the first year after a mastectomy.

- Joined a research team in 1962 for a five-year sociological study of personnel and dying patients as the only woman and nurse in a male-dominated competitive group of researchers

- Formulated the Transition Services Model of Practice

- Codeveloped, with faculty member Ruth McCorkle, the Oncology Transition Services graduate program within the Department of Nursing at the University of Washington.

RIGHT
Quint Children
Jeanne (far left) and her sisters
Diana and Patricia, 1929

BIOGRAPHICAL INFORMATION

BIRTH

Jeanne C. Quint was born December 9, 1919, in National City, CA, at the home of her maternal grandparents.

PARENTS

Jeanne's father, John Edwin Quint, was born in Oshkosh, WI, in 1885. His ancestry in North America dated back to the pre-Revolutionary war times. He joined the Navy at age 21, learned the trade of a machinist, and made the Navy his life's career. John spent a year with the fleet that President Theodore Roosevelt sent around the world. Jeanne's mother, Marie Lydia Wade, was born in Sioux Falls, SD, in 1889. Marie attended nursing school at St. Joseph's Hospital in St. Paul, MN, and received her license to practice in 1912. She chose to do private duty nursing, which, at that time, meant moving into patients' homes during the duration of their illness. A move to San Diego led Maria to meet her future husband, John, at a dance. They married in 1917 and first lived in National City, CA. Later, they settled in a home that they built in San Diego, where John was assigned to a large naval base for much of his time in the Navy.

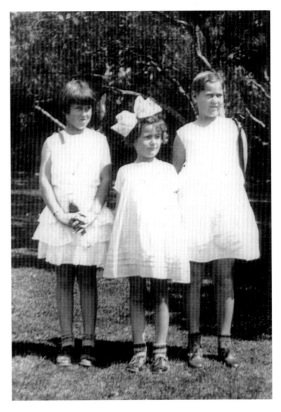

FAMILY

Jeanne, the oldest of three girls, was considered her mother's "golden egg." She was born in California at the home of her maternal grandparents when her father was stationed at the naval base in the Philippine Islands. Jeanne always received good grades throughout school and pursued a variety of interests, from mathematics to painting. She wanted to continue her education in finance, but the Depression financially prohibited it. Nurses' training was a more practical and much less costly alternative. Because she was only 17 years of age when she graduated from high school and the required age to enter nursing school was 18, Jeanne stayed at home and attended San Diego State College for one year. Jeanne entered a hospital nurses' training program in San Francisco after turning 18. Her sister Diana, after graduating from college, taught music in the San Diego schools and never married. Patricia, Jeanne's youngest sister, went to secretarial school, married, and had three children. She died in 1956 of a brain-stem hemorrhage while eight months pregnant with her fourth child. The career choices available for women at that time were nursing, teaching, or secretarial, and the Quint family had one of each.

CAREER PATH

Jeanne experienced a complex intertwining of personal and professional transitions that led her to become a nurse scientist. Her first decade in nursing was marked by completion of her studies at St. Luke's Hospital training school in San Francisco in 1941. She passed the state

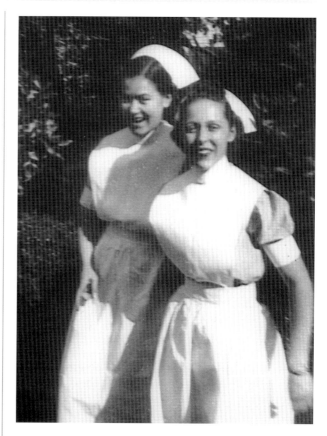

board examination to become a registered nurse and worked for two years at the San Diego County Hospital as a staff nurse and 27 months in the Army Nurse Corps in the South Pacific Theatre during World War II. The GI Bill allowed her to study for two years at Oregon State University for her bachelor's degree.

FRESNO GENERAL HOSPITAL SCHOOL OF NURSING

In 1948, Jeanne took a teaching position at Fresno General Hospital School of Nursing in California, where she remained for the next five years. During this time, she met and married her first husband. After two years, she found it necessary to admit him to a state mental hospital for paranoid schizophrenia. By 1953, she made the painful decision to leave the marriage for the sake

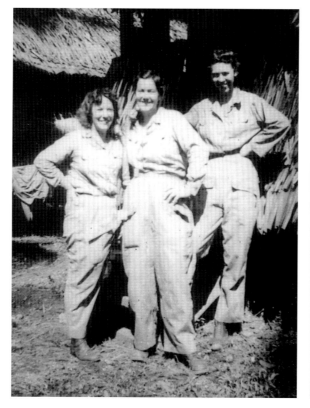

ABOVE
Jeanne Quint (left) and Jane
Wright (right) after capping
St. Luke's Hospital, School of Nursing
San Francisco, CA
1939

LEFT
Army Nurses
Jeanne Quint (center)
Milne Bay, New Guinea
April 1944

JEANNE QUINT BENOLIEL

RIGHT
Jeanne Quint
1955

BELOW
John E. Quint (father), Jeanne
Quint, and Marie Quint (mother) ·
Jeanne receiving her master's
degree from UCLA
June 1955

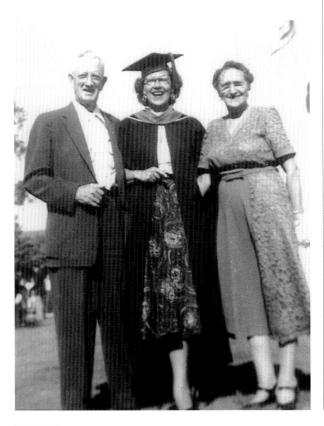

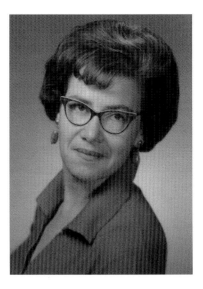

of her life, which slowly was being destroyed by the dynamics surrounding her husband's illness.

UNIVERSITY OF CALIFORNIA, LOS ANGELES

Jeanne relocated and enrolled in a graduate study program in nursing at the University of California, Los Angeles (UCLA), received a master's degree in 1955, and joined the faculty of the UCLA School of Nursing for the next four years. During this time, certain crises occurred in Jeanne's personal life: a serious depression following her divorce, the sudden death of her sister in 1956, her mother's major surgery, her father's death from gastric cancer in 1958, and her own "scare" of finding a breast lump that required a biopsy, which, although negative, created an enormous fear of cancer. These critical family events led Jeanne to think more deeply about the meaning of death and dying and how people adapt to periods of crisis and change. She began to ask questions and seek answers that would help her to understand more about life's transitions. These events in her personal life significantly altered the direction of her professional life and gave her a focus that she continued to pursue throughout her professional career.

Although Jeanne enjoyed teaching, she was looking for a new challenge. This led her to enroll in an experimental research postmaster's program for nurses, which was being conducted at UCLA from 1959–1961. That choice initiated her shift into a research career and the role of coinvestigator of a two-year, funded research study in the adjustment processes of women during the first year after a mastectomy. This study was conducted at a time when secrecy about cancer was commonplace. Information control by healthcare professionals and others was discovered to be a powerful factor in women's opportunities to talk about what it meant to have cancer and how it was affecting them and their families. Jeanne recognized the role nurses played in the communication process.

Nursing has always been concerned with the care and comfort of the patient, and I submit that the professional nurse can play an important part in helping both the patient and the physician cope with the difficult problems which a cancer diagnosis brings . . . she can help the patient face reality by letting him talk about his cancer when he is ready to do so, and she can be an important communication link between the patient and the physician. (Benoliel, 1965, p. 131)

The study showed that living with the identity of being a person who has cancer and facing a life of uncertainty and possibly a painful and difficult death is not an easy task and often a lonely one. This study also taught Jeanne new ways of thinking about phenomena in the world and means for understanding these phenomena in systematic ways, as well as recognizing the difference in perspective of practitioners and investigators.

UNIVERSITY OF CALIFORNIA, SAN FRANCISCO

In 1962, Jeanne moved to San Francisco, and, for the next five years, she worked as a research sociologist on a study of dying patients and hospital personnel headed by Anselm Strauss, faculty member at the University of California, San Francisco (UCSF). The purpose of the study was to describe the kinds of death that hospital personnel face in their work and to see how staff members react to and cope with various aspects of death. The effort was an early attempt at understanding dying as a human behavior within the context of a hospital. For Jeanne, this experience was her entry into the world of sociology and the complexities of field research. During those five years as the only woman and nurse on a research team, her awareness of the "marginal" world increased. As the dying patient study grew to completion, Jeanne realized that a doctoral degree was a necessity if she was going to stay in academia. She enrolled in the doctoral program in nursing at UCSF, and, in 1969, she was the first nurse to be awarded a DNSc degree. After graduation, Jeanne joined the faculty at UCSF. She used the multiple meanings of death as a framework for a course, "The Threat of Death in Clinical Practice."

Jeanne became active in the human rights movement in 1956 while living in Los Angeles. This continued to be a concern of hers in San Francisco. She willingly spoke out on civil rights issues and chose to join a picket line in support of such things as equality in housing. Dancing, especially folk and square dancing, provided Jeanne with a social outlet that she enjoyed and put her in touch with people other than her nursing colleagues. While living in San Francisco, she was active in the Unitarian Church, attended seminars and conferences at Esalen, and joined an organization called San Francisco Venture, which was a group of "people who were searching." It was during this time that Jeanne met her second husband, Bob Benoliel.

UNIVERSITY OF WASHINGTON SCHOOL OF NURSING

Jeanne married Bob in 1970 and moved to Washington where she joined the nursing faculty at the University of Washington. Her continued interest in the

To bring about changes in nursing practices is a difficult matter. Indeed, the problem is truly a question of changing attitudes which are based on deeply entrenched cultural and subcultural values and which underpin, at least in part, the basic nurse identity.

BENOLIEL, 1965, P. 132

BELOW
Jeanne and Bob Benoliel
Fall City, WA
1975

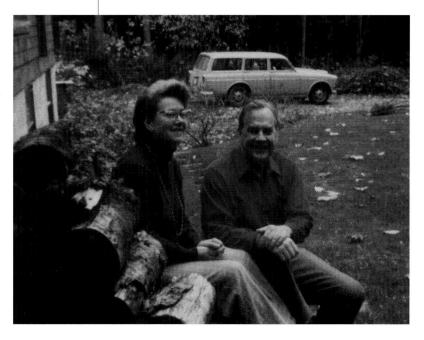

JEANNE QUINT BENOLIEL

The process of preparing this summary caused me to reflect on the relationship between past and present and between present and future. I was reminded once again of two points worth repeating. All knowledge and accomplishments in cancer nursing today were built on the ideas and activities of earlier generations of nurses. Affiliation between older and younger generations of people—in this case nurses—is a vitally important connection in the collective transformation of society toward a humane existence for all human beings.

BENOLIEL, 1989

importance of supportive environments for people undergoing major transitions was applied to the formulation of the Transition Services Model of Practice. This model formed the basis for a training grant that she and Ruth McCorkle received from the Division of Nursing in 1977–1980. With this grant, she and Ruth developed a unique community-based graduate program, Oncology Transition Services, within the School of Nursing. This highly acclaimed program was extended for several years, and, between 1977 and 1989, 53 nurses graduated from the program. Many of these nurses have filled the leadership roles in oncology nursing.

Although the period of time between 1975 and 1980 was wrought with progressive pain of arthritis for Jeanne, successful hip surgery in 1981 offered her renewed energy to pursue her professional endeavors. She was appointed as the first Elizabeth Sterling Sould Professor at the University of Washington, a title she held until her retirement in 1990.

Jeanne spoke of each of her professional experiences as building blocks in her professional development as a nurse scientist. She best expressed this in the following statement.

Along the way, each of us encounters individuals who are influential to our personal growth as human beings. These significant individuals can be other nurses whose ideas stimulate our own, key patients with whom we have contact over long periods of time, and key persons whose choices and actions were critically important to the care of patients and families. (Benoliel, 1998)

Publications from both of her first two research projects led to many invitations to give papers, workshops, and consultations. She assumed an active role in both regional and national nursing activities, such as the California League for Nursing, numerous positions with the California Nurses Association, American Nurses' Association, American Nurses' Foundation, American Cancer Society, International Work Group on Death, Dying, and Bereavement, and the governing boards of Sigma Theta Tau and the American Academy of Nursing. As her work became known, so did her reputation as a nurse scientist. The National Cancer Institute used Jeanne's research expertise on a number of site visits. She accepted invitations from Israel and Japan to serve a visiting professorship. All of these additional professional opportunities fostered Jeanne's understanding of the practical and political realities of conducting research on sensitive subjects, increased appreciation of the difficulties women in health-related profession face world wide, and expanded her intellectual horizons.

RECOGNITION

Jeanne began receiving awards early. In 1941, as top student in her nursing class at St Luke's Hospital School of Nursing in San Francisco, she received the Monteagle Award of $250 to be used in advanced education. In 1959, she received a two-year fellowship of $4,000 per annum from the National League of Nursing to study in a two-year experimental research training program at UCLA. A Predoctoral Nurse Fellowship from the Division of Nursing in 1967 facilitated her doctoral study at UCSF. In 1972, the UCLA Alumni Association awarded her the Professional Achievement Award, and, shortly thereafter, she was elected as a Fellow in the American Academy of Nursing. The American Cancer Society recognized her work with their Distinguished Service Award in 1984. She was honored with the Excellence in Teaching Award at the University of Washington, the Distinguished Merit Award by the International Society of Nurses in Cancer Care, and the Distinguished Researcher Award by the Oncology Nursing Society (ONS). Jeanne received honorary degrees in 1989 from the University of San Diego and in 1993 from the University of Pennsylvania. These awards and honors are just a few of the many that stand to recognize Jeanne's many contributions as a nurse researcher, educator, and mentor. In the year 2000, Jeanne received one of nursing's highest recognitions when she was designated a Living Legend by the American Academy of Nursing. All of nursing applauded Jeanne when she received this singular honor.

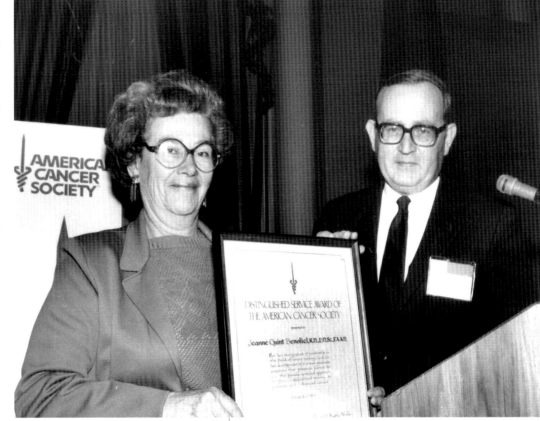

ABOVE
Jeanne receiving the American Cancer Society Distinguished Service Award from Dr. Gerald Murphy 1984

RETIREMENT

Following retirement, Jeanne continued to provide her expertise in other arenas. She helped to establish a new doctoral program when she was a professor at Rutgers University; she was a consultant at the University of Pennsylvania; and she was a member of the Ethics Task Force of ONS. Jeanne cut short her three-year teaching contract at Rutgers when her husband became ill, first with prostate cancer that required a series of radiation treatments and then with heart prob-

JEANNE QUINT BENOLIEL

BELOW
Jeanne with her cat, Morris

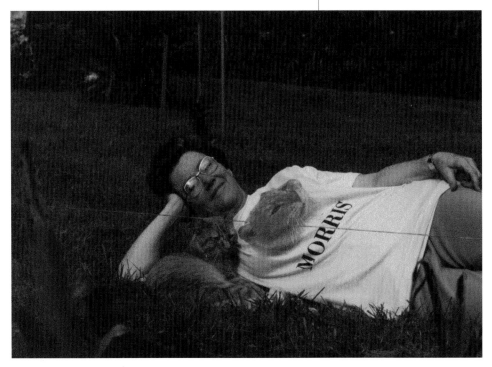

lems that required bypass surgery. Jeanne's own health problems with hypertension and glaucoma began to compromise her health as well. Jeanne described the years between 1992 and 1994 as ones in which each other's (her and her husband's) health became their primary responsibilities. Fortunately, with time and Jeanne's good nursing care, they both regained their strength and stamina, which allowed them to carry on a full and satisfying life together. However, such chronic conditions as osteoporosis, cataracts, and hypertension continued to reduce their energy levels and made them extremely selective in what they chose to do. Their home in the country, located an hour from Seattle, provided them with the peace and quiet they both enjoyed. Their major social focus has been their nine great-grandchildren, most of whom live in the area. In the fall of 1999, Bob died in a Seattle hospital following surgery. Jeanne remains in their home and keeps active as her health permits. She occasionally meets the "Old Guard," who are the former faculty members at the University of Washington, and continues to serve on the editorial boards of *Cancer Nursing*, *Western Journal of Nursing Research*, and *Omega*.

Jeanne is selective about accepting invitations to speak. A few special events that she has chosen include the Clare Dennison Lecture at the research conference to honor her colleague Jean Johnson, who was retiring from the University of Rochester School of Nursing, the Heritage lecture at the University of Arizona College of Nursing, and the research conference on Chronic Disabling Conditions. She also wrote a paper on the *Twentieth Century Change and the Death Movement* sponsored by the Society for Care of Children and Families Facing Illness and Death in Athens, Greece. Jeanne continues to participate in the International Workgroup on Death, Dying, and Bereavement, a group of colleagues that she has associated with since the inception of the workgroup in 1974.

When asked which event or award stands out as the most exciting and rewarding for her, Jeanne is quick to describe "Jeanne Quint Benoliel Celebration Day" that was held at the University of Washington in May of 1989. Ten of her former students presented papers describing their research or practice activities and spoke of the role Jeanne played in their lives. Following the students' presentations, Ruth McCorkle, her professional colleague, spoke of the influence that Jeanne's work has had on nursing and nursing science. Jeanne said, "To know you have had a positive impact on those who follow in your footsteps is a reward that is truly immeasurable."

SUMMARY

Jeanne's prolific professional nursing career as a researcher spans more than 35 years. It began in 1961 with a longitudinal study of the adjustments women experience the year following a mastectomy. Her findings indicated that living with uncertainty about when and how death may come became an important facet of these women's lives. Patterns of personal as well as familial adaptation were heavily influenced by unspoken fears about death. This study was conducted at a time when secrecy about cancer was commonplace. Subsequently, Jeanne joined a research team at UCSF in a sociological study of hospital personnel and dying patients. These early endeavors provided the foundation for her ongoing contributions in the influence of life-threatening illnesses on patients, families, and healthcare providers. Her inquiries consistently focused on two inter-related themes: the impact of catastrophic life events on personal identity and environmental influences on the nature and form of major life transitions involving the threat of death and dying.

REFERENCES

Benoliel, J.Q. (1988). Jeanne Quint Benoliel. In T. Schorr & A. Zimmerman (Eds.), *Making choices, taking chances: Nurse leaders tell their stories* (pp. 15–22). St. Louis: Mosby.

Benoliel, J.Q. (1989, December). *From research to scholarship: Personal and collective transitions*. Paper presented at the American Cancer Society First National Conference on Cancer Nursing Research, Atlanta, GA.

Benoliel, J.Q. (1995). Jeanne Q. Benoliel. In B. Nevidjon (Ed.), *Building a legacy: Voices of oncology nurses* (pp. 47–60). Boston: Jones and Bartlett.

Greene, P. (Ed.). (1984). Cancer nursing profile: Jeanne Quint Benoliel, RN, DNSc, FAAN (1984–1985). *Cancer Nursing News, 3*(4), 4.

Benoliel, Jeanne Quint, interview by Judith Johnson, February 1999.

JEANNE QUINT BENOLIEL

SELECTED WRITINGS
ABSTRACT

Title: An Exploratory Study of Women's Adjustment Following Radical Mastectomy*
Staff: Lulu Wolf Hassenplug, Principal Investigator
         Jeanne C. Quint, Project Director

The study was designed to examine the adjustment required of women during the first year following mastectomy. The sample consisted of 21 women who had surgery at a medical center hospital. Included were all women who had mastectomy during a 6-month period of hospital field work and showed no sign of metastases except axillary nodes at the time of surgery. Six received medical care from private physicians, and the remainder were supervised by the medical resident staff. Data were collected by participant observation in the hospital by two nurses who provided nursing care in collaboration with the nursing staff. The same two nurses conducted home interviews with participants at 2 weeks, 6 weeks, 3 months, 6 months, and 12 months postsurgery. Only one woman withdrew after the first home interview. These interviews were audiotaped and transcribed for subsequent analysis. The findings showed the women meeting one of two outcomes. They either did not survive the year or began a living pattern marred by concerns about when they might die. With wound healing and physical wellbeing as standards, the women could be separated into three groups. Six women faced an uncertain future despite clear wound healing and apparent recovery. Thirteen faced an uncertain future combined with physical complications of various sorts. Two underwent rapid physical deterioration and died during the year. A major difficulty identified by all the women was obtaining valid information about what was happening to them and being able to talk to someone about their real concerns. Across the year they became progressively isolated with their "disease". Inadvertently, the nurse interviewers came to function as the only people to whom they could talk about their concerns and fears.

*   This study was supported by NIMH Grant M5495 and jointly sponsored by the School of Nursing and the Department of Surgery, School of Medicine, University of California, Los Angeles, for the time period 1961–1963.

Note. From "An Exploratory Study of Women's Adjustment Following Radical Mastectomy" [Abstract] by L.W. Hassenplug and J.C. Quint, University of California, Los Angeles. Supported by NIMH Grant M5495, 1961–1963.

THE IMPACT OF MASTECTOMY, *AMERICAN JOURNAL OF NURSING* (1963)

Disfigurement and cancer are words that individually carry a negative connotation in our society. Some women personally come face to face with both simultaneously through having a breast removed for malignancy.

—

The participants gave us their views of the three basic changes which this operation initiates. First, it precipitates a period of shock and unexpected events. Second, it leaves a change in bodily appearance. Third, it mars the future by the prospect of shortened life and the possibility of slow, painful death.

The first look at the incision frequently comes as a tremendous shock. It strikes most forcibly when the woman stands before a mirror and looks at herself. In describing her feelings one woman said, "I'll never forget the first time I saw it. Not the lack of what you used to be but the horrible scar was what got me down. Oh, this horrible purple piece of flesh up here! I'm very self-conscious about it, and I don't want anyone to see me. I had to dress it the first day at home and that was pretty rough, too."

—

The period of upset and agitation was often prolonged by such things as delayed wound healing, some other complication, or by having radiation therapy.

—

Most women expressed surprise at the amount of pain and discomfort, the marked fatigue, the slow healing of the incision, the swelling of the arm, and jittery feelings. They expected to be feeling better by four months and frequently were amazed to find themselves going through a phase of letdown and continued exhaustion.

—

It was common to find that family and friends were interested and concerned at first but soon expected the patient to return to normal.

An all encompassing problem, harder than dealing with the deformity, is the question, often not said aloud: What is my future? It is as though almost anything that happens can trigger the thoughts: Am I going to die? When? How?

You wonder why these things have to happen. I don't know. Things come to your mind. Maybe the kids have something they don't want to tell me. Maybe they know something.

⌇

For many, changes in physical signs and symptoms took on new meaning and were used as cues for testing the future.

⌇

These women described what it was like to undergo a treatment, mastectomy, which not only did not guarantee a long and happy life by removing the cancer but also inflicted them with the stigma of being half a woman, a not too happy prospect in a breast-conscious society such as ours. For these women there was a central core of loneliness, the key element being that they had few if any outlets for talking about those things which most concerned them. They were stuck with two relatively taboo subjects: a defeminizing disfigurement and the prospect of dying.

⌇

Is Any Woman Immune

That breast cancer and mastectomy are potent subjects for women in our society is illustrated by what happened to the study staff, all of whom were women. There were two major consequences for the interviewers.

Because the interviews contained a great deal of personal and emotionally laden material, we had to come to terms in some way with our own feelings about cancer, loss of a breast, and death, not to mention a tremendous sense of inadequacy in the situation. We had to face the fact that we, too, were frightened and wanted to run away. We found it extremely difficult to permit others to talk about disturbing events when our own fears were rising.

The second consequence was that some of the women who were interviewed became worse. Some, in fact, did not survive the first year. It was hard enough to talk to those who at least superficially were recovering, but it was sometimes agonizing to watch someone go downhill, eventually to die. It was this experience which was the hardest to bear.

Even the secretaries who typed the interviews found themselves caught in the intensity of highly emotional experiences.

To continue the study, we interviewers found that we had to talk to each other to get our own reactions and feelings out in the open. Even so, it was difficult to go on. We found, just as did the women in the study, that most persons won't permit talk about upsetting things. It became apparent that professionals, like laymen, found such talk intolerable. We interviewers, too, found ourselves in a lonely position.

As one listened to these women postoperatively describe their lives in transition, one was struck by the lack of professional guidance offered to them. The major problems they faced alone, not because family and friends lacked concern or did not try to help, but usually because the latter were also caught in the tragedy and were made impotent by it.

It became evident that, as a by-product of the study, the interviewers were providing the opportunity for these women to ventilate about matters which were generally forbidden in their everyday social contacts, both familial and otherwise. They were permitted to let their hair down about what it is really like to live with a mastectomy. The interviewers, in turn, paid a price for this experience; eventually we had to face the thought: This could happen to me.

Articles in lay magazines have made it well known that breast cancer is the most common form of cancer in women. It is estimated that one woman in 20 can expect to have it. In spite of publicity to the effect that early diagnosis and mastectomy will cure, there is no guarantee of this. Breast cancer is a capricious disease as professionals and patients know. What woman is immune from the question: Will this happen to me?

It is not surprising to note that most women function to minimize their personal identification with the problem and make use of such protective devices as avoiding the topic altogether or keeping discussion of the operation at a sociable level.

One would expect to find that nurses, most of whom are women, act much the same as women in general, and this is indeed so. In fact, one would be surprised to find otherwise since this group not only have access to privileged information about postmastectomy recurrence and survival statistics but also have given care to women with breast cancer in varying stages. Those who have seen death and suffering from breast cancer cannot so easily minimize personal identification with it.

Nurses' Reactions

It is true that there are individual women who are able to cope with this fearful problem admirably and to offer sustenance and support to postmastectomy patients . . .

These women are unusual, however, and are rarely available to the majority of those who undergo this operation. After mastectomy, most women are not yet ready to talk while still in the hospital. Even if they were, they have little access to nursing personnel except for brief contacts centered on procedures and physical tasks. That nursing personnel do not openly initiate discussion about mastectomy and its personal meanings is the rule, not the exception.

It is not difficult to understand, however, that nurses use such a device to protect themselves from a woman's situation which they would find hard to handle. It makes even more sense when one recognizes how little preparation most nurses have had for coping with such a problem.

A student nurse recently made this response when she was asked if she had seen many women with breast cancer, "Yes, and I don't like it. It's one thing I can't stand. This sounds silly but I think I could stand to have a leg off rather than a breast because of the idea of being disfigured."

She was asked if she had taken care of many of these women. "I think my nursing care is poorer here because I relate it to myself. I find it hard to talk, and these people are ones who need it so much. They do need a lot of care. I'm sure if I had to have a mastectomy, I'd never get used to it."

It was appropriate to say to her, "Don't feel bad. You're not alone," but one was reminded immediately that many women are going it alone with their mastectomies.

It is no small thing to have a breast removed for cancer, and adjustment to living with the change comes slowly. Most surgeons cannot offer the kind of sustained support which these women want. Perhaps this is not the surgeon's job, for what can he know of what it is like to be a woman?

For nurses to accept responsibility in this problem, however, they must be willing to forego the practice of saying, "That's the doctor's responsibility," and be willing to face a problem which offers no easy solutions. Perhaps the first step for many is to agree with the student nurse who said, "I think my nursing care is poorer here because I relate it to myself."

Note. From "The Impact of Mastectomy," by J.C. Quint, 1963, *American Journal of Nursing, 63*(11), pp. 88–92. Copyright 1963 by Lippincott Williams & Wilkins. Excerpted with permission.

AWARENESS OF DEATH AND THE NURSE'S COMPOSURE (1966)

This study, begun in 1961, was an exploratory investigation of dying as a usual hospital event—a social phenomenon which involves many different persons (patients, families, and a variety of health workers) and which takes place under varying sets of conditions. It was our purpose to describe the kinds of death which face hospital personnel in their work, and to see how the staff react to, and cope with, the various aspects of death. We were not solely interested in death as an end-point and the circumstances under which it occurred, but in understanding social interaction around and in the dying situation. Both the study design and the methods chosen for data collection reflect two basic characteristics of this investigation: its exploratory nature, and the temporal component of the problem. We were studying a dynamic, not a static situation.

A study of this sort has both theoretical and practical implications and is useful, therefore, both to practitioners and to those concerned with abstract ideas. By describing the practices presently observed to take place around dying patients, one initiates the opportunity for open dialogue among health professionals concerning these practices and whether or not changes are needed. From a theoretical viewpoint, a study of dying within a given context—the hospital—can be useful for identifying recurrent patterns of social interaction among different groups of persons when the crucial identity of one of the interactants is at issue. For those interested in process, the study can also serve to clarify the developmental aspects of interaction and the interplay between social interaction and social structure as conditions vary through time.

Discussion

Analysis of the social structure and work styles of hospital wards with high death ratios is useful for detailing the kinds of work problems which nurses commonly encounter when they care for dying patients, the circumstances under which these problems take place, and the strategies which develop for managing those aspects of dying which are troublesome for the nursing staff. The analysis confirms the hypothesis that a distaste for death, demonstrated in this society, carries over into hospital culture and is reflected in the behaviors of hospital staff toward dying patients—most notably in their withdrawal from talking openly with dying patients about the process of dying. Inspection of the avoidance strategies used by nurses shows that many of these strategies are no different from those utilized by persons in middle class society for minimizing personal involvement with individuals who are dying or whose diagnosis is more or less synonymous with dying.

A comparative analysis of two "high death" wards, one stressing recovery and the other comfort till death, shows clearly that an emphasis on recovery goals can quite successfully mask the presence of death and protect the staff much of the time from the impact of dying. The nurses in intensive care units often do not define dying patients as dying because their work situation permits them to maintain this definition, but nurses in other parts of the hospital do essentially the same thing. That is, they tend to see and hear those things which tell them that the patient will get well but they avoid those facts which tell them that he is probably dying. If

JEANNE QUINT BENOLIEL

the nurse does not define the patient as dying, she does not have to deal with him on that basis, and since she has been trained to focus her attention and energies on life saving practices, she finds few rewards in caring for the dying patient. Inasmuch as hospital work on most services is organized around recovery goals, no matter how unreal they may be, the nurse has little difficulty in keeping herself uninformed of the true "death expectations" of many patients. As a consequence, a patient often cannot behave as though he were dying or even express his fears about the possibility.

That dying is a difficult task for nurses is illustrated by the composure strategies developed on a cancer research ward for controlling those aspects of dying which are likely to be maximally upsetting if they get out of hand: conversations with patients and families and provision of painless comfort during the final period of life. It is the nursing staff, more so than the medical staff, which bears the brunt of this task. Many problems arise because most doctors and nurses do not talk directly to patients about the possibility of dying, nor do they talk to each other about what is happening, or they think about dying as a social phenomenon and plan accordingly. Often their differences in interpretation of the patient's dying status can lead to misunderstandings of one another's actions and to frustrations which spread throughout the entire staff. Needless to say, there are important consequences for patients when physicians and nurses are unable to cope with the interactional aspects of dying, and dying patients are prevented from making decisions about their final days.

Note. From "Awareness of Death and the Nurse's Composure," by J.C. Quint, 1966, *Nursing Research*, *15*(1), pp. 49–55. Copyright 1966 by Lippincott Williams & Wilkins. Excerpted with permission.

TRIBUTES

I first became familiar with Jeanne's writings when I was in graduate school at the University of Iowa in the late 1960s. I was studying to be an oncology clinical nurse specialist, and cancer was equated with a death sentence. Jeanne's publications "The Impact of Mastectomy" and "The Nurse and the Dying Patient" were extremely helpful to me as I was developing my skills in talking with patients about cancer and its implications. Jeanne had married and changed her name to Jeanne Q. Benoliel in 1970. I made contact with Jeanne in 1973 while I was a student in the Mass Communications doctoral program at the University of Iowa. I was working on a problem statement as the basis of my dissertation and needed feedback to see if I was expressing myself clearly. I sent Jeanne a copy of my paper and she responded quickly with constructive feedback. She encouraged me to contact her again, and, subsequently, she agreed to be a reader for my dissertation proposal. We maintained contact throughout my studies, and I arranged to meet her briefly at one of the national nursing conferences in St. Louis in 1974. Although I only had about 30 minutes with her, she reinforced the importance of the work I was trying to do, she acknowledged the stressful nature of the work for providers, and she seemed genuinely interested in my career. Upon graduation, I very much wanted to work more closely with Jeanne. It was my dream to have regular contact with her and to develop educational programs to prepare nurses for the stress they encounter in working with patients with cancer and their families.

As I was about to defend my dissertation, I wrote to Jeanne at the University of Washington to see if they had a faculty position available. I interviewed, and, to my surprise, I was hired. Of course, I wasn't hired to teach oncology, but I thought the opportunity offset looking for the ideal job in oncology. At that time, there were no specialty programs, and I was assigned to teach undergraduate senior nursing students about leadership. As a part of that course, I had to supervise seniors with their last clinical rotation. I was only two weeks into the program, and I was in hot water. I had worked with a student about discussing dying with a woman scheduled for an adrenalectomy for breast cancer ablation. The student talked frankly with the patient, and the patient seemed very grateful for the opportunity to discuss her fears with the student. I debriefed the student and checked with the patient to be sure that the student had not provoked unnecessary anxiety. The student charted her encounter and left the unit. When the surgeon made rounds, all hell broke loose. He wanted to know who the student was and who her instructor was. His belief was that talking about death would somehow interfere with the patient's trust in him and that the operation would be unsuccessful. He believed that the patient's state of mind made a difference in her recovery. He immediately called the dean at the School of Nursing, and the dean called Jeanne. Of course Jeanne tracked me down. She asked

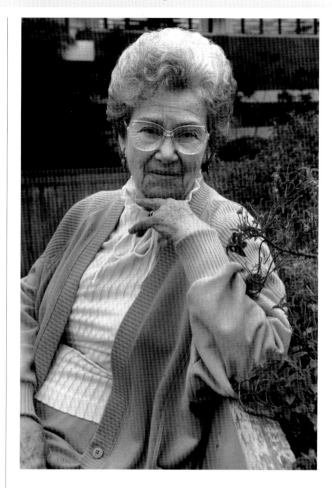

ABOVE
Jeanne Quint Benoliel

JEANNE QUINT BENOLIEL

what happened in a calm and reassuring voice. After I conveyed what the student had done under my supervision, Jeanne said, "Well what are you going to do about it? The surgeon never wants you in his hospital again." I really thought I had done something wrong. That day Jeanne taught me one of the most important lessons of my life. She told me that this was a man who I would continue to work with for many years and that I had to go to him, apologize for not meeting him sooner, and introduce myself. The meeting had to be in private and at the end of the day when he was tired, preferably on his feet all day after surgery and after rounds. She said to simply tell him that I wanted to be a member of the team and what would he recommend in the future about talking with his patients. Tell him that I need his advice and that I want to teach students to help, not interfere, with patients' recovery.

This is only one example of the wise consult Jeanne has given me over the years. I worked with her from September 1975 through December 1985. We consciously divided our efforts in most of the activities we were associated with. She was a leader at the American Cancer Society, so I put my energies into the Oncology Nursing Society. Jeanne worked hard for the Academy of Nursing and the International Work Group on Death, Dying, and Bereavement. I became involved with the International Society of Nurses in Cancer Care and the American Society for Psychosocial and Behavioral Oncology. Together, we accomplished what neither of us could do as one. We started the first community-based oncology nursing graduate program, "Oncology Transition Services"; we started the first nonmedical pre- and postdoctoral nurse research training program in "Psycho-social Oncology"; we developed two of the first outcome measures to be used with patients with cancer, the "Symptom Distress Scale" and the "Enforced Social Dependency Scale"; and we had consistent federal research funding for our research program during 10 years as coinvestigators.

Jeanne's writings remain inspirational to me. She is one of the most prolific scholars I know, and her contributions remain true to practice today. Jeanne once told me that she writes for herself. I have never met anyone who works as hard as Jeanne. She has high standards for herself and everyone who works with her. She loves excellence in others—a great tennis match, an unforget-table opera, a well-acted movie, and a delicious meal. She helped me to strive to be the best I could be. She remained available to listen whenever I needed to talk, but she also respected others and their privacy and wanted everyone to value her privacy. Jeanne has strong values about personal choice, integrity, and human dignity, including one's right to suffer. Jeanne's personal and professional life was changed dramatically when her sister died during childbirth. This important event crystalized her commitment and passion to devote her life's work to the nurse's role in the care of the dying. She has remained a true champion of patient and family rights and as a voice for the vulnerable. She believes nursing is primarily women's work—although she probably has taught more male nursing and medical students than any other nurse researcher I know.

Jeanne has a great sense of humor. She participated in the annual competitive skits at the Western Research meetings. One of her most memorable roles was as a "lady of the evening" when she wore a bright red dress with black accessories. Jeanne also is known for her outrageous earrings, and some believe that to be a true qualitative researcher, the earrings are a part of the dress code. Jeanne's responsiveness to my ideas early in my academic career development greatly influenced me, especially the way I interact with people who want to learn from me and contribute to practice. I was fortunate to work with her and to have her as my friend and colleague. We all need heroes in our lives. Search and you can find one.

Ruth McCorkle, RN, PhD, FAAN

Professor
School of Nursing
Yale University
New Haven, CT

Jeanne Quint Benoliel has forged the career paths of countless cancer nurses, including myself. My first encounter with Jeanne was in 1975 when I knocked on the door of her faculty office. After explaining the purpose of my master's thesis, I asked Jeanne to serve on my reading committee. Not one to mince words, she responded, "Why do you want me to be on your committee?" What popped out of my mouth was quite unexpected. I said, "Because I want the best!" No truer words have ever been uttered by a lowly graduate student in the presence of a world-renowned scholar and nursing pioneer.

I learned during the next dozen years while working with Jeanne that she expects no less of her students than of herself. She challenged the clarity of my thinking and writing as a fledging doctoral student. As a postdoctoral fellow under her tutelage, she taught me the historical roots and scope of the emerging field of psychosocial oncology. Jeanne introduced me to the rigors and rewards of conducting qualitative inquiry in her graduate class on symbolic interactionism and grounded theory development and guided my first efforts at conducting participant observation in the field.

Two of Jeanne's early publications were influential in my decision to enter oncology nursing and to conduct research on the personal meaning of cancer. Her seminal paper, "The Impact of Mastectomy," not only described the emotional, social, physical, and existential effects of this disfiguring surgery on the lives of women, but it explicates for future generations of nurse scientists the conflict generated by the juxtaposition of two conflicting identities: clinician and researcher (Quint, 1963).

Jeanne revealed how she and her research colleague endeavored to set boundaries between their roles as clinicians, giving direct care to the women in the study, and their roles as data collectors and participant observers. Moreover, she described what it is like as a researcher and woman to come to terms with feelings of inadequacy, fear, and loss, as many of her research participants experienced progressive disease, a steadily worsening state, and, in some cases, death. This classic publication should be mandatory reading for all nursing graduate students who aspire to enter a career in research.

I consider another early paper by Jeanne to be her most scholarly and profound publication. "Institutionalized Practices of Information Control" (Quint, 1965) influenced the direction of my dissertation research, and it continues to guide my thinking about the ways people with cancer strive to obtain information during situations of information deficiency or ambiguity. At the core of this manuscript is the affirmation that cancer nursing is, above all else, a social transaction. Care providers shape the behavior of people with cancer by adhering to institutionalized tactics that regulate patients' access to privileged information about the severity and prognosis of their disease. Consequently, often lacking objective information, people with cancer may experience anxiety and uncertainty as they struggle to make sense of and give meaning to the potentially life-threatening illness.

I wanted the best, and I got it. Few people have done more to influence the delivery of informed, humanistic, and ethical care to people with cancer and to assert each patient's right to self-determination than Jeanne Quint Benoliel. It remains one of my highest honors to brag to others that Jeanne was my former professor. Jeanne has taught all of us what it means to be a cancer nurse and what it takes to make a difference in the lives of people with cancer.

Mel Haberman, RN, PhD, FAAN

Associate Dean for Research and Professor
Washington State University
College of Nursing
Spokane, WA

REFERENCES

Quint, J.C. (1963). The impact of mastectomy. *American Journal of Nursing, 63*(11), 88–92.
Quint, J.C. (1965). Institutional practices of information control. *Psychiatry, 28*, 118–132.

Professional papers and effects of Jeanne Quint Benoliel are located in the archives at the Nursing History Center at the University of Pennsylvania in Philadelphia, PA. Additional information and papers used during the preparation of this text are archived at the National Office of the Oncology Nursing Society in Pittsburgh, PA.

NORMA OWENS, AB, AM, RN, EdD
Leader in Cancer Nursing Education and Internship Opportunities

"The nurse listens, gently questions and listens some more during the initial evaluation . . . If we listen, the patient will disclose their philosophy of life, living and death from their own personal perspective of 'what is.'"

— Norma Owens

SIGNIFICANT CAREER CONTRIBUTIONS

- Coedited, with Rosemary Bouchard-Kurtz, *Nursing Care of the Cancer Patient*, Fourth Edition, 1981

- Received the Sword of Hope Award for 25 years of continuous volunteer service with the New York Division of the American Cancer Society, 1985

- Worked for 30 years as a faculty member in the Division of Nurse Education at New York University, 1955–1985, with major contributions to and the further development and sustainment of the Internship in Oncological Nursing program

- Professor Emerita of Nursing in the Division of Nursing at New York University, 1985

BIOGRAPHICAL INFORMATION

BIRTH AND DEATH

Norma Francell Speese was born on January 14, 1924, in Thedford, NE. She died in October 1996 in Kansas City, MO.

PARENTS

Norma was born to Hannah Rachel Rosetta Meehan and Charles Speese.

FAMILY

Norma's doctoral dissertation is dedicated to specific family members, her mother and four siblings, who had cancer. She noted two sisters and a brother as being cured of cancer: Ava Geraldine, uterine cancer; Kenneth Fahe, mediastinal cancer; and Allison Elaine, cervical cancer. She also dedicated the dissertation in memory of her brother, Clifford Benjamin, who died of a brain tumor in October 1961. Whether she had other siblings who were not affected by cancer is unknown. Her mother died of a renal tumor in 1966.

Norma was married to James "Jimmy" H. Owens, a mechanic. They had no children. For many years, Norma and Jimmy made their home in Staten Island, NY. Norma was an avid gardener who took great pride in the flowers that she grew.

CAREER PATH

Norma graduated from the Perth Amboy General Hospital School of Nursing in Perth Amboy, NJ, in 1950. Her first professional position after graduation was as a staff nurse at the hospital. Staying on at the hospital of a diploma school after graduation was fairly common at that time. Many hospitals identified staff recruitment as a major benefit of having a hospital-connected school of nursing. Hospitals often recruited students by suggesting that staying on for a year after graduation was an expectation in recognition of the expenses that a hospital incurred in maintaining its program. This program also helped to keep tuition and expenses considerably lower than those that students would encounter at college-based programs. Although it is not known whether this was the case at Perth Amboy General Hospital, it is certainly a good possibility.

In 1952, Norma earned a bachelor's degree from the San Francisco State Teachers College in California. She then worked as a staff nurse at the U.S. Public Health Service Hospital in Staten Island. Her interest in cancer care was stimulated during this time. In 1955, Norma joined the faculty of the Division of Nurse Education in the School of Education at New York University

(NYU). Norma began her teaching career at the instructor level and continued this affiliation for 30 years. During those years, she was part of numerous important programs, initiating some and adding new dimensions to others. Considering today's educational requirements, the fact that Norma began teaching other students when she only held a bachelor's degree is amazing. She did, however, begin work on a master's degree at NYU's School of Education in late 1956.

In 1958, Norma enrolled in NYU's doctoral program, the beginning of a 10-year journey. Two scholarships, a Title II Federal Traineeship Grant and a Sigma Theta Tau Scholarship Award, helped to fund Norma's education. Norma wanted to study personality changes, that resulted in major body image or function changes in patients who had undergone cancer surgery. She considered studying patients who were undergoing mastectomy and those having surgery resulting in ostomy. She decided that for her study population, she wanted patients who had head and neck cancers because the facial defects following surgery for these cancers were immediately visible and could not be hidden. Norma believed that because this patient population had to face disfigurement, they were different than patients in whom body change could be covered with clothing. Norma felt that patients responded differently, had a different outlook, and could have recuperated better if the defect could be covered.

Dr. Martha E. Rogers chaired the sponsoring committee for Norma's dissertation, "A Study of Personality Changes in Males With Severe Facial Deformity During the First Six Months of Adjustment After Radical Surgery for Cancer." Norma's test-retest study design followed a sample of 109 men from their first hospitalization for radical cancer surgery and at three postsurgical test periods. Patients inside and outside of the study began to ask to see "the talking nurse," a title of respect that Norma deserved as she developed her psychosocial skills. In a 1987 interview, Norma noted that the patients talked and she listened. It did not matter what they wanted to talk about; most just wanted to be heard. She recalled that while one man paced when he talked, she paced with him. He was worried about his home and invalid wife and expressed concern about his ability to continue caring for his wife as he had preoperatively. In her teaching, Norma stressed the importance of listening at every possible opportunity. Following Dr. Rogers' philosophy and model of nursing practice, Norma stressed the individual as a whole person, facilitating integration of this model into nursing care approaches.

INTERNSHIP IN ONCOLOGICAL NURSING

Between 1955 and 1970, Norma was involved with the Internship in Oncological Nursing program, an NYU educational program with a clinical affiliation at the James Ewing Hospital, which was located adjacent to the Memorial Hospital for Cancer and Allied Diseases (now Memo-

The purpose of this investigation was to determine personality changes in adult male patients who had radical surgery for cancer of the head and neck and to determine the relationship of these changes to job status, family status and verbal communication status. A further purpose was to determine the extent to which these patterns changed over a six month period.

OWENS, 1968

Unless you as an individual (I-me-myself) have been faced in reality with a diagnosis of cancer, not one person can truthfully say what they would do, how they would react to this news, or what societal factors of living would impinge on decisions for self.

OWENS, 1985, P. 43

NORMA OWENS

BELOW
Norma Owens and Judi Johnson

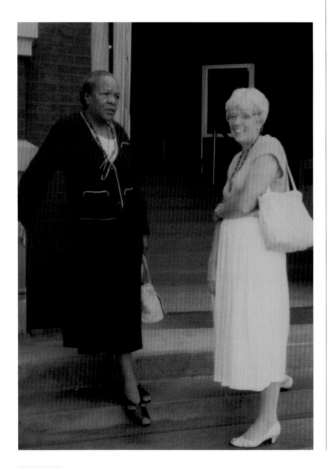

rial Sloan-Kettering Cancer Center). The New York City government ran James Ewing Hospital, an aging teaching center. Memorial Hospital was a voluntary hospital. The structure and titling of buildings and programs during this time is slightly confusing. A 1953 report on the internship program described the Memorial Center for Cancer and Allied Diseases as including Memorial Hospital, James Ewing Hospital, the Sloan-Kettering Institute for Cancer Research, the Tower Out-Patient Department, and the Strang Prevention Clinic.

The administration of the facilities was separate, and each hospital had its own nursing staff. The medical staff was the same for both hospitals. As Norma phrased it, "If you had money, you went to Memorial; if you were poor, you went to Ewing." The medical care was outstanding at both: "You could watch the medical teams finish rounding at Memorial, come out the backdoor, and enter Ewing's to begin rounds there—the same physicians."

Patient distribution at James Ewing Hospital was organized by anatomic site, with units for head and neck, breast, gynecologic, and genitourinary cancers. Two units served as the inpatient beds for the Sloan-Kettering Institute for Cancer Research, a 36-bed chemotherapy services unit and a 30-bed unit for metabolic and other clinical research activities. A chronic shortage of nurses made it difficult to provide adequate care. The idea of collaborating with NYU's Department of Nursing Education was raised in hopes of bringing students to the unit who would be able to assist in providing care and who might stay on as staff. This was the beginning of the internship program.

The description for NYU course 141.133, Internship in Oncological Nursing, states, "This is a New York State approved program of university level, combining professional theory with practice in the clinical situation. Since cancer is one of the major health problems today, this course is meeting a dynamic social need, and has a futuristic outlook toward long-term planning in the field." The internship was a four-credit course, with a five-day, 40-hour workweek. The New York City Department of Hospitals paid students a stipend to cover living costs. They also received laundering of their uniforms and two meals per tour at token cost. (The maximum cost was $0.35 per day.) The Sloan Foundation funded the program, and the City of New York paid the nurses' stipends. Funding varied and increased during the years of the program, but the money was substantial for the time. In 1961, for example, the total support from the Foundation and the city was $160,000. An additional $5,000 came from Lenk-Wallace Scholarship Funds to support student tuition.

The initial director of the program was NYU faculty member Rosemary Bouchard. Norma was an instructor. The initial class had three participants, and Norma observed that the program was "slow to get off the ground." The full-time demands of the program plus the negative connotation of cancer care most likely contributed to the slow start. Faculty purposefully used the term "oncological" instead of "cancer" to try to avoid the negative connection. Clinical rotations included all major treatments, with faculty drawing from their own areas of clinical expertise in dividing the didactic content.

A 1957 medical administration report outlined the ideal table of organization for nurses in the two units as 39 registered nurses, with at least 20 nurses' aides. Current staff at that time consisted of only 20 registered nurses, one of whom was the supervisor for both units, 6 practical nurses, 14 nurses' aides, and 4 nurse interns. The report states that the nurse interns "... are RNs who spend three hours a week in class rather than on the wards." Continued emphasis on the shortage of nurses in cancer care is seen in many reports from this time period. In a later 1957 communication between NYU's School of Education Dean George D. Stoddard and Dr. Rogers, Dean Stoddard reported meeting with Dr. Cornelius Rhoads and other physicians and administrators at the Sloan-Kettering Institute. Dr. Stoddard wrote that the "... gist of the conversation was the thought on their part that the program of internship for nurses should be stepped up, made more appealing, and pointed to an enrollment of perhaps 40 persons. (It now enrolls 17.) It was implied that the continuance of the program on a five-year basis beyond 1958 would depend on a new and more exciting plan. The teaching potential is not fully developed. The city and other units need the graduates." Dean Stoddard charged Dr. Rogers with interpreting these generalizations, noting that even the course sheets "... are indeed drab."

In 1959, another aspect of the internship program, Clinical Study in Oncological Nursing, was initiated. This program built on the ongoing internship program by offering an additional postinternship year of study at the undergraduate level for registered nurses. The added year offered a stipend equal to a starting nurse's salary and was seen as an opportunity to develop in-depth skills in specific areas of cancer care and to allow further study toward a bachelor's or master's degree.

Norma and her fellow faculty members worked hard to develop the program even further over the next two decades. A new, attractive blue and white recruitment folder was developed. The number of nurses began to increase, allowing the chemotherapy unit to increase its operational capacity. Pay levels were adjusted and increased for all city-employed registered nurses in late 1957 and 1958, and approaches were planned to address the difficulty nurses encountered in finding appropriate and affordable housing. Norma and her coworkers studied nurses' motivation to participate in the internship program and to practice in the research setting in general. One report stated, "The cases seen and cared for on research services are conceded to represent a unique educational opportunity medically and from the nursing point of view. This attribute of our services should be exploited to its utmost. Even if we lose a well-trained nurse,

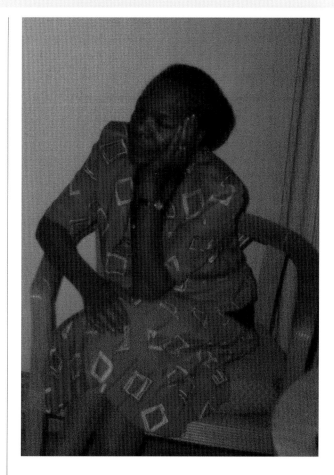

ABOVE
Norma Owens

I do remember that every year she arrived at school laden with armfuls of exquisite, colorful Chinese chrysanthemums that she grew at her home on Staten Island. I also had a garden, so we would talk about the exotic mums. It was then that I had a glimpse of Norma under circumstances removed from the university, with its multitudinous duties and obligations. For a moment, Norma was herself, as her beauty reflected in her brief, tender, spontaneous interactions with the stunning flowers. Time stood still, and space was filled with her love for all living things. Those were moments that left me in awe of the woman whom I had studied under and worked with for so long and of whom I understood so little.

DOLORES KRIEGER, RN, PHD
PROFESSOR EMERITA NURSING SCIENCE
NEW YORK UNIVERSITY
SCHOOL OF NURSING

we may profit when she exhibits her knowledge and training to other nurses who may then desire to come here."

Over time, the internship program gained size, strength, and value. Additional personnel who felt it was a primary reason why the ward's census increased noted the value of the program. The nurses also were seen as advocates who referred other staff members. Additionally, the program began to recruit foreign nurses who had to be proficient in English. Recruiting foreign students posed new challenges for the faculty in orienting these nurses to equipment, procedures, and the parameters of the Nurse Practice Act. After the first five years of the program, Rosemary Bouchard left NYU to pursue a doctoral degree. Norma was named acting director of the program and later director. During these years, Norma collaborated with Edith Wolf, education director at Memorial Hospital, in planning and reporting program activities. Another very close colleague was Inga Thornblad, an NYU faculty member who taught in the internship program and who was active with Norma in American Cancer Society activities. Inga was diagnosed with breast cancer and asked Norma to help her continue teaching for as long as possible. With Norma's help and Inga's perseverance, Inga taught class on the day she died.

Between the initiation of the program in 1955 and its termination in 1976, approximately 640 nurses from 34 countries participated. Although many students were not able to stay on after the year-long program, several did. Overall, the program was seen as extremely valuable in helping to change the image of oncology nursing, in improving the care delivered to patients, and in addressing recruitment problems. After such a success story, it must have been very difficult for Norma and the other faculty members to see the program come to an end. Changes in the administration and operation of the James Ewing Hospital, the centralization of education and nursing services under the Memorial Hospital umbrella, and general alleviation of the nursing shortage at that time contributed to this decision.

NEW YORK UNIVERSITY

After the internship program closed, Norma continued at NYU in graduate education and as director of the master's program in biophysical pathology. In 1970, she received a Woman of Achievement Award from the Brown Bombers Association of Staten Island, NY, and a Certificate of Recognition from the New York City Board of Education for giving eight years of dedicated service to the Staten Island School Board.

From 1974–1979, she served as an assistant administrator within the division of nursing at NYU, followed by an appointment as a full professor in 1975. During all of these years, Norma supported and mentored students, providing a needed liaison with minority and foreign students.

She served on a variety of committees at the university and in the New York City area.

Norma's meritorious service to education and community was well recognized in the remaining years of her career. In 1979, she received the Meritorious Great Teacher Award from the NYU Alumni Federation and University Board of Trustees, followed in 1980 by a Citation Award commemorating 25 years of teaching and service from the School of Education, Health, Nursing, and Arts Professions at NYU. In 1981, she received a similar Citation Award from the Alumni Federation of NYU.

Norma was coeditor with Rosemary Bouchard-Kurtz of the fourth edition of *Nursing Care of the Cancer Patient*, published in 1981. The intent of the first publication in 1967 was to provide a text for the internship program students. The need for this book in other nursing centers and by nurses across the country became obvious, and successive editions aimed to include newer and broader information as it became available. Norma authored or coauthored nine chapters, including subjects easily recognized as her specialties—"Psychosocial Components of Cancer Nursing," "Nursing Care of Patients With Head and Neck Tumors," and "Nursing Care of the Patient With Terminal Cancer."

AMERICAN CANCER SOCIETY

Norma was an active volunteer with the American Cancer Society (ACS) throughout her career. She developed a professional network that planned activities and provided local and regional education programs. Norma served as a member of the Nurses Advisory Committee in 1980 and 1981 and was editor of the proceedings of the Seventh and Eighth Inga Thornblad Oncology Nurse Conferences (1980–1981), *Coping With Realities of Terminal Cancer: The Nurse, The Patient, The Family*. ACS recognized the contributions Norma made by giving her a Woman of Achievement Award in 1972 and the Sword of Hope award in 1980 for 25 years of continuous volunteer service in the New York City division.

Nursing care of THE CANCER PATIENT

Rosemary Bouchard-Kurtz
Norma Speese-Owens

FOURTH EDITION

LEFT
Norma was coeditor with Rosemary Bouchard-Kurtz of the fourth edition of Nursing Care of the Cancer Patient, published in 1981.

BELOW
Norma was editor of the proceedings of the Seventh and Eighth Inga Thornblad Oncology Nurse Conferences (1980–1981), Coping With Realities of Terminal Cancer: The Nurse, The Patient, The Family.

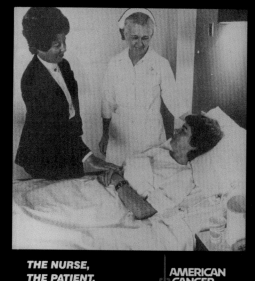

THE SEVENTH and EIGHTH
PROCEEDINGS 1980-1981
INGA THORNBLAD ONCOLOGY NURSE CONFERENCE
COPING WITH REALITIES OF TERMINAL CANCER

THE NURSE,
THE PATIENT,
THE FAMILY....

AMERICAN CANCER SOCIETY

SUMMARY

Norma Owens was a very private person. We know little about her early life, and she brought little of her personal life to her professional work. She was a dedicated nurse and an exemplar to others, as indicated in the reports about the internship program. It is unusual today for a nursing educator to stay as long Norma did at one facility and to devote so many years of effort to one program. Norma was the right person at the right time for an important project. Norma identified the internship program as her most prized accomplishment. She stayed in touch for many years with nurses who completed the program, several of whom came to her retirement dinner. Norma always was interested in hearing what they were doing, what they had accomplished, and how they were continuing to improve the care of patients with cancer. In 1977, Norma attended the International Council of Nurses meeting in Japan, a final professional opportunity. Four former students attended, and Norma enjoyed reminiscing about their times together at the James Ewing Hospital.

Norma Owens died in October 1996 in Kansas City. She leaves a special legacy of dedication to a major program. She helped hundreds of nurses to launch careers in oncology nursing, instilling in them a sense of excitement about oncology nursing, the need to listen to patients, and the importance of continually staying abreast of new information.

REFERENCES

Bouchard, K.R., & Owens, N.S. (Eds.). (1981). *Nursing care of the cancer patient* (4th ed.). St. Louis, MO: Mosby.

Owens, N.S. (Ed.). (1985). *The seventh and eighth Inga Thornblad oncology nurse conference. Coping with realities of terminal cancer: The nurse, the patient, the family.* New York: American Cancer Society.

Owens, Norma, interview by Susan Baird, 1987.

Papers from the archived materials of Norma S. Owens, Oncology Nursing Society, Pittsburgh, PA.

Papers from the archived materials of Edith S. Wolf, Oncology Nursing Society, Pittsburgh, PA.

SELECTED WRITINGS
COPING WITH REALITIES OF TERMINAL CARE (1985)

Unless you as an individual (I-me-myself) have been faced in reality with a diagnosis of cancer, not one person can truthfully say what they would do, how they would react to this news, or what societal factors of living would impinge on decisions for self.

There are many facets to decision-making processes about patient and family welfare during an illness. They must be helped to believe that they are an integral part of that decision-making process. Three patient rights assume importance during such periods. First, the right to know: What is the diagnosis, plan of therapy (and why), and the patient prognosis. Second, the right to appropriate therapy: The patient may well say, "Level with me; tell me the truth." They can demand that no 'unusual' measures be taken; they have the right to refuse usual modes of treatment. Thirdly, the patient has the right to informed consent, the right to decide in final judgement what therapy should be and how far it goes before they say, "Stop here." As indicated by Kübler-Ross, when hope is gone, the patient no longer needs or asks for external help.

During the phase of terminal illness, close observation, knowledgeable assessment, open communication and careful evaluation of the patient and family are basic ingredients for professional intervention. The foundation of nurse action rests on basic tenets of:

1. Accept patient/family feelings as being a normal response.
2. Help the patient/family to make peace with reality.
3. Detailed information is not always the best; stop where and when the patient stops–listen!
4. The patient and family can perceive only what they are capable of assimilating at any given moment, especially when the prognosis becomes negative for life.

These tenets include nurse recognition and understanding of the level of readiness to know; anxiety about knowing; denial against knowing; expectations of what must be known for their future.

Approaches to nursing care also include a clear perspective as to whether the patient is existing, surviving or living with the cancer diagnosis. Existing with cancer has negative connotations of helpless hopelessness. There are visible behaviors of letting go or decathecting from loved ones and life, however slowly until the inevitable end. Surviving cancer infers that the person has had no evidence of disease (N.E.D.) for 3–5 or more years. However, there is always the unspoken fear in the mind that a recurrence is possible. This fact is its own kind of nightmare. If cancer does recur, the psychological reaction is far more devastating than living through the original diagnosis.

NORMA OWENS

An oncology nurse specialist epitomized this philosophy when she wrote,

". . . My energies are exchanged with both the patient and family. I intervene; there is a comfort in my presence as a knowledgeable, compassionate and caring advocate nurse. . . . When I now contemplate death, I find great comfort in the special profession I have chosen."

Living with cancer has a positive aura of hopefulness, even though that attitude may eventually become hope for death. The essence of patient hope and belief is: "Yes, I know I still have cancer but, perhaps, just perhaps in my lifetime, the scientists will find that long-sought-for cure of my dilemma. Meanwhile, I will fight to stay alive and live each day to the full. So much needs to be accomplished for me and all of us in this situation. Our orientation is toward a hopeful future for each of us, it hangs in the glory and beauty of a new sunrise for that future." There is a special kind of joy and hope in the beliefs and actions of these patients that not one of us can fully realize unless, we too, have lived their experience of cancer.

The nurse experiences professional growth and new levels of autodiagnosis – 'know thyself'– when caring for the person with cancer. Very often, it is the patient who does the teaching. Beyond the development concepts of age perspectives, of culture, ethnicity or religious beliefs, the reality of humanness is the most important for the nurse to understand when caring for the person who is terminally ill and dying of cancer. An oncology nurse specialist epitomized this philosophy when she wrote, ". . . My energies are exchanged with both the patient and family. I intervene; there is a comfort in my presence as a knowledgeable, compassionate and caring advocate nurse. . . . When I now contemplate death, I find great comfort in the special profession I have chosen."

Note. From "Life Perspectives and the Dying Process" (pp. 43–44) by N.F. Owens in *The 7th and 8th Inga Thornblad Oncology Nurse Conference: Coping With the Realities of Terminal Care*, 1985, Atlanta, GA: American Cancer Society. Copyright 1985 by American Cancer Society. Excerpted with permission.

DOCTORAL DISSERTATION (1968)

Introduction

The purpose of this investigation was to determine personality changes in adult male patients who had radical surgery for cancer of the head and neck and to determine the relationship of these changes to job status, family status and verbal communication status. A further purpose was to determine the extent to which these patterns changed over a six month period.

A sample of 109 adult males of the greater metropolitan area of New York were included in the test-retest study as they were admitted for the first time to hospital for radical surgery for cancer of the head and neck region. The Cattell 16 Personality Factor Questionnaire (Forms A and B) was the instrument selected for measurement of presurgical norm scores at admission for comparison with the 3 postsurgical test periods at 5 days after surgery during hospitalization, and at 8 weeks and 6 months after being discharged.

The obtained data was analyzed 1) for the total sample and 2) by the three social status classifications of job (employed, unemployed, retired), family (lives-with-family, lives-alone) and ability to communicate (verbal, nonverbal).

Chapter VI. Discussion of Findings in Relation to Implications for Nursing and Recommendations for Further Research

In recent years, the various health findings have broadened their concept of "patient care" to include the areas of in-depth rehabilitation and recognition of the individual as a community person within his total environment for living and functioning. Nursing leaders, educators and researchers have often led the way in efforts to assume the social responsibility of viewing health services beyond the traditional concept of "the sick." Findings of the current investigation add emphasis to the need to move beyond conventional attitudes and practices, to advance contemporary functioning with normal people who seek help in times of difficulty with their health.

Implications for Nursing

The person entering, or returning to a health agency for follow-up, spends many precious hours awaiting his turn for "the" decision. Empirical observations of the clinic setting indicated that conversation between patients or between patients and personnel, tended to be minimal, factual to the immediate situation and/or superficially impersonal. Discussions with patients during their clinic visit revealed that these persons are fraught with anxieties, fear of the unknown, ignorance due to unanswered questions and the desire to talk with someone whom they trust and believe possesses a genuine interest in their welfare as a whole person.

The question was raised as to the possibility of more effective use of time spent in clinic. Here is a captive audience for the nurse to practice rehabilitative teaching, to discuss individual health problems with the patient and, thus, ascertain areas of misunderstanding, eliminate ignorance of the body and its functions, foster mental health with recognition and identification of effects of therapy on the person's future and, on the basis of the foregoing, to exercise nursing intervention in relation to restorative measures toward acceptance of physical deviance, social responsibility to self and reality-oriented goals toward a unified existence as a human being with purposeful activities to fulfill.

Research data demonstrated that needs of patients in clinic differ between the initial, pre-admission visits and the post-therapy appointments that will continue—even once a year—for the person's lifetime. The first 6 months, and possibly more, appear to be critical in assisting the patient in his search for direction and social acceptance, in his struggle to re-affirm his own integrity as he attempts to face the realities of life.

The person entering, or returning to a health agency for follow-up, spends many precious hours awaiting his turn for "the" decision.

Here is a captive audience for the nurse to practice rehabilitative teaching, to discuss individual health problems with the patient . . .

NORMA OWENS

Originating from findings of the investigation, recommendation is made here (1) to inaugurate a pilot study to determine feasibility of nurse instruction of patients on a group basis during clinic hours, (2) to initiate controlled experimental research to determine the therapeutic effectiveness of nurse intervention through patient instruction and/or (3) to institute health teaching by the nurse for patients during clinic hours, separating the pre-admission group from the follow-up group of patients.

There are also strong implications for additional nursing research, with the unemployed and retired groups of subjects, in particular. These two groups evidenced patterns of personality change and behavioral response to therapy over the first six months that frequently was at great variance from the data obtained for the total group—and other subgroup data.

Another factor that bears implications for nursing and nursing research that was not clearly delineated by the current investigation is the multitude of problems created for the geriatric person, particularly during hospitalization. The contemporary term given to the point-in-question is "the dehumanization process" that may occur, especially with this age group, during hospital confinement. It is suggested that much of this error is directly related to nurse attitude and concurrent practices at the patient bedside. Although these persons may be "grateful" that surgical intervention did not result in more severe handicaps than those he has, yet the geriatric adult also has an inherent right to the dignity of his manhood, his integrity as a person and the rights, privileges and obligations that the role implies. The elder subjects in the study became sober, group-dependent and subdued but they were also significantly suspicious, apprehensive and tense. Did these factors cover the significant scores of practical, controlled, alert poise? Has this person "gone-into-hiding" in his nurse-expected roles in a situation already too difficult to cope with: to what extent has the nurse compounded his difficulties of rehabilitation?

An aspect specific to nursing that aroused interest of the investigator was the families of the patients, their relationships with the patient and effectiveness of the family role in progression of the patient toward successful rehabilitation. Implications for both nursing research and nursing intervention can readily be ascertained in relation to direction of social responsibility and interaction with therapeutic goals on a long-range basis in assessment, promotion and maintenance of health.

Observations of and conversations with subjects in follow-up clinic instigated questions regarding effects of prolonged association with a health agency after therapy. There are a number of postulates that could be investigated in relation to nursing responsibility—and the dangers of irresponsibility—toward the patient in the clinic setting and community activities. For example, there is need for long-term nursing research into prolonged psychological invalidism, adaptation to loss of valued sources of gratification, of extent of destruction and integrity as a person and fulfillment of life goals, and effects thereof, on the patient and his family.

Medical statistics indicate that malignancies are now the second leading cause of death from disease and that persons so affected are increasing in number each year. It is a recognized fact that there is a growing "shortage" of nurses, to the extent that it is of nationwide concern. Each factor affects the other. The available number of active nurses must be utilized in the most efficient manner possible in order to provide adequate care for the patient undergoing treatment for cancer; the majority of these patients is composed of the very young and the elderly.

Patterns of disease and means of therapeutic intervention are directly correlated with a growing body of scientific knowledge, and practical application of that knowledge, for the health and welfare of mankind. Problems of the patient with cancer are a realistic part of the changing health picture. Over one million citizens now living have been cured of cancer. A significant population that is even larger is composed of the survival group that is well five years after therapy. It is the cured and survival person, as well as the "hopeless case," who require knowledgeable intervention and care by nurses combining with other disciplines. "The primary aim of nursing service is to provide care of the type needed, and in the amount required, to those in need of nursing care . . . (this can only be accomplished) when nurses in education and in service recognize their interdependence and actively collaborate to achieve the ultimate aim of both—improved nursing care.[1] "Education's translation into service is nursing's social goal."

Education of nurses is rapidly becoming differentiated for two specific groups: the professional nurse and the technical nurse. Each group has clearly defined knowledges and skills for clearly defined levels of performance in a variety of clinical settings. The educational preparation of the nurse should determine her responsibilities in care of the patient. Studies of nurses repeatedly stress that job satisfaction follows significant utilization of the nurse's career preparation. Attention to differentiation of nursing practice has been both minimal and misdirected. Staffing patterns of health agencies strongly suggest that nurse roles are determined more on the basis of immediate expediency than according to nature and level of preparation. Promotion of health is hindered by the traditional assumption that the term, registered nurse, is applicable for utilization by society as one level of nursing role. Such practice has resulted in what is now recognized as a need for change. This with a central core of change in attitude toward health practices and a four-pronged plan of action affecting (1) education of nurses, (2) significance of the nursing role, (3) agency utilization of nursing staff and, of greatest importance, (4) results as measured by the ultimate recipient in promotion of health for society, the patient; specifically for this investigation, the person with cancer.

Changing patterns of nurse education necessitate changing patterns of attitude and utilization within the clinical agency. The task of changing attitudes must be confronted. Freedom to achieve excellence must be within the province of all who nurse. Employing agencies must provide a climate in which each person can develop his potentials to the utmost. The role of the clinical setting in conducting research and demonstrating appropriate staffing organization and re-training of nurses would have significance and applicability on a nationwide scale.

Investigations in the science of nursing add to nursing's theoretical structure and concomitantly provide the knowledge that can be translated into practice. Their significance is not only to nursing but to others concerned with people. Most important of all, today's investigations in nursing science foretell a future of scientific evolution in nursing that must underwrite our social responsibility—our commitment to human kind.

References

American Nurses Association. (1965, December). Position paper on nursing education. *American Journal of Nursing, 65*, 106–111.

Rogers, M. (1964). *Reveille in nursing*. Philadelphia: F.A. Davis Company.

Rogers, M. (1967). *Nursing science: Research and researchers*. Paper presented at the Annual Conference on Research and Nursing. Division of Nursing Education, Teachers College, Columbia University, New York.

Note. From *A Study of Personality Changes in Males With Severe Facial Deformity During the First Six Months of Adjustment After Radical Surgery for Cancer* (1968), by N.F. Owens. Unpublished doctoral dissertation, New York University, New York.

TRIBUTES

Norma Owens was my advisor when I was in the master's program at New York University (NYU). Throughout my course of study, her guidance always was diligent, accurate, and thoughtful. Norma frequently nominated me for and helped me to be selected for membership in professional organizations.

When I joined the nursing faculty at NYU in 1977, Norma served as a mentor to me. She helped me to negotiate the system, which enabled me to achieve the goals I had set for myself.

I still can remember how well she handled the traineeships for students, particularly the scholarships she administered to the minority students in the Division of Nursing. She was a strong advocate for the rights of all people.

Once, when Norma was on sabbatical, I was assigned to teach one of her courses, "Nursing Strategies for the Adult and Aged." She willingly gave me the materials she had used for the course and provided valuable resources. She even contacted me during her sabbatical to be sure everything was going well.

Norma loved parties. She always helped to plan parties for the Division of Nursing. She made sure that the division always was decorated for the various holidays, often paying for the decorations herself.

Norma was generous and kind. May her soul rest in peace.

John Phillips, RN, PhD

Associate Professor
Division of Nursing
School of Education
New York University

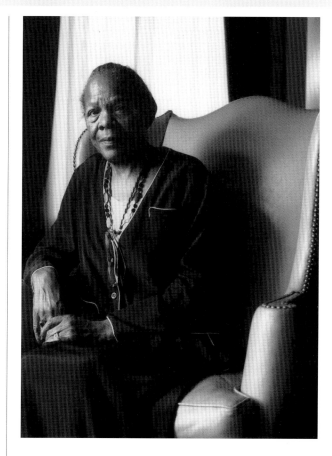

ABOVE
Norma Owens

I first met Norma at James Ewing Hospital when I was working under Inga Thornblad, my "master teacher," while I was taking the course "Apprentice College Teaching." Inga was Norma's dear friend and colleague in the oncology nursing program and, along with Rosemary Bouchard-Kurtz, helped to teach that program. When I met her, Inga had breast cancer and had endured several surgeries and some chemotherapy, so Norma often was my "master" when Inga was unable to come to work. Inga and Norma were incredible women and real colleagues and collaborators. Norma supported Inga's desire to work until she died. Both women mentored me as I learned to teach. I also learned a great deal about oncology nursing, especially in pediatrics. Inga and Norma helped me to locate resources, plan lessons, and find slides, and they spent hours listening to me teach and critiquing me. Norma's critiques were straightforward and tough. I learned a lot from Norma and Inga, not only about teaching, but also about humanity.

When I joined the faculty at New York University, Norma was one of the first people to really welcome me. Norma knew my husband, who had been a student in the James Ewing program, and remembered him well. She remembered me from my earlier years as a student teacher. She invited us to visit her home on Staten Island every late spring/early summer for a cookout, and it was always a treat. Norma was a good cook, and her husband, Jimmy, was a great host with lots of good stories. Norma was "house proud" and loved her home and garden.

Norma was a special mentor to African American and international students in the nursing department. The Ewing program attracted a large number of students from countries outside of the United States, so Norma had to learn a lot about Immigration and Naturalization Service regulations. She was nurturing and supportive when the inevitable homesickness happened and when cross-cultural conflicts arose. As one of the few African American women on the faculty at the university, she made a real effort to be available to help both nursing and non-nursing African American students. Norma also administered a small fund for students who needed urgent temporary loans.

Norma was proud of her heritage, which also included Native Americans. I remember two pictures in her office, one of a black man playing a guitar and one of a slave cabin with people standing around the door. She also had a wonderful wooden rocking chair in her office, which I suspect offered real comfort to students in trouble.

I remember a story about Norma keeping copies of her dissertation chapters in the freezer of her refrigerator because when her first house burned down, she lost all her work and had to start over again. I cannot vouch for the truth of that story, but every doctoral student in my era kept the latest copies of their dissertations in their refrigerators.

Joanne King Griffin, BS, MA, PhD

Associate Professor
Division of Nursing
International Student Coordinator
School of Education
New York University

Professional papers and effects of Norma Owens are located in the archives at the National Office of the Oncology Nursing Society in Pittsburgh, PA.

JANET LOUISE MCKENZIE LUNCEFORD, RN, MSN
Leader in Cancer Nursing Education and Clinical Practice

"The nursing care of patients with acute leukemia is challenging because . . . the care of these patients can often be extremely complex and can tax all the nurse's skills and ingenuity. It can also be enlightening because the nurse will be constantly amazed at the adaptability, courage, and strength that these patients display . . ."

— Janet Louise Lunceford

JANET LOUISE MCKENZIE LUNCEFORD

SIGNIFICANT CAREER CONTRIBUTIONS

- Created the *milieu management* program for adolescents with leukemia

- Directed the nursing care of patients in the first Life Island isolators and Laminar Air Flow Rooms

- Implemented a work-study program in cancer nursing for nursing students

- Developed a post-master's fellowship contract program in oncology nursing

RIGHT
McKenzie Children
Janet Louise and brothers,
Robert, Kenneth, and Dean
1935

BIOGRAPHICAL INFORMATION

BIRTH

Janet Louise McKenzie was born on January 17, 1925, in Blawnox, PA.

PARENTS

Janet Louise was the second of four children born to James E. McKenzie and Hilda R. Tillotson. Both of her parents were born and raised in Pennsylvania. Her father, James and his brother, were raised by an uncle. Little is known about his background except that he came from a Scottish heritage. James worked as a steel worker all of his life. Hilda completed one year of nursing school in Warren, PA. During that time, she met James, left school, and married the following year. Hilda's maiden name, Tillotson, has been traced back to a 17th-century English heritage.

FAMILY

The McKenzies first settled in Pennsylvania, where Louise, the name her family used to call her, and her three brothers were born. Hilda was a homemaker, played piano, and was active in church activities. Louise described her childhood years as normal. She recounted a time in second grade when she dressed up like a nurse for a party and told her teacher that she wanted to be a nurse. Because she was always the tallest child in her classes, she often was teased, especially during her grade school days. The principal, who was a tall lady, told her that when she walked, she always should look up at the tall trees or telephone poles. Louise always has remembered this admonition.

Louise's oldest brother, Dean, began to draw early in life and encouraged Louise to pursue her interest in drawing as well, which she has continued to do over the years. Dean attended a fine-arts high school, and after a tour of duty in the Marines, studied at the Chicago Art Institute and became a commercial artist. He became known for his artwork, especially his pastel landscapes. He had four children with his first wife.

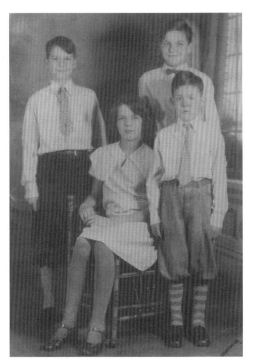

He died of lung cancer in 1998. Louise speaks affectionately of her brother and has a number of his paintings displayed in her home next to those she has painted. Louise's younger brother, Robert, died in an accident at age 20. Her other brother, Kenneth, had a rare debilitating disease, periarteritis nodosa, which led to his death at age 29. Louise has remained close to his wife and two children. Her niece, Susan, chose to become a nurse, and Bobby, her nephew, went into the lumber business.

The McKenzie family made several moves during Louise's childhood, first to Massillon, OH, then to Pennsylvania, to Buffalo, NY, and finally back to Massillon. These moves were precipitated by Louise's father's need to find employment. Louise spent her first two years of high school in Buffalo and finished school in Massillon. Louise's mother, who required medical intervention for malignant hypertension for several years, died of a stroke at the age of 42. Louise was 17 at the time and ready to graduate from high school. Her father remarried shortly after and moved the family to Cleveland, OH. Louise enrolled in nursing school in Akron, OH. James' second wife, Agnus, died in 1971, and he died the following year because of complications from a hip fracture.

CAREER PATH

Louise attended a three-year training program in nursing at Akron Hospital in Ohio. She has many memories of her student nursing days, including 12-hour shifts that were split between morning and evening assignments, a tour of duty in the diet kitchen, and wearing pink uniforms, which led to students being called "pinkies" during their pediatric rotation. Because of her love of working with children, Louise sought a job at the Children's Hospital in Akron following graduation. After a year, she and two friends moved to Columbus, where they enrolled at Ohio State University for two quarters, with the intent of obtaining their bachelor's degrees. When her friends prematurely left school, Louise did likewise and moved near relatives in the Pittsburgh area, where she took a staff nurse position at the Women's Hospital. Agnus Campbell, a nursing supervisor, encouraged Louise to return to school and complete her degree. Taking her advice, Louise obtained her bachelor's degree in nursing at the University of Pittsburgh in 1951. Following graduation, Louise was offered the position of Instructor in Surgical Nursing at Presbyterian Hospital in Pittsburgh.

AIR FORCE

In 1952, Louise entered the Air Force as a first lieutenant and was assigned to Maxwell Air Force Base in Montgomery, AL. She worked as a staff nurse in the hospital's general medical/

ABOVE
J. Louise McKenzie
Student nurse
Akron Hospital, 1944

BELOW
J. Louise McKenzie
Graduation
University of Pittsburgh
1951

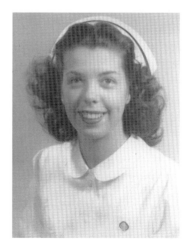

JANET LOUISE MCKENZIE LUNCEFORD

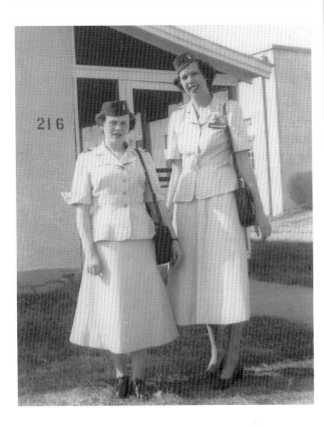

surgical unit. Here she met Sigmond A. Lunceford, who was a senior pilot and judge advocate general officer in the Air Force. Sigmond had been a bomber pilot during World War II and was a graduate of the University of Alabama Law School. Louise and Sigmond married in the summer of 1953. Shortly thereafter, he was reassigned to a base in Texas, which necessitated them living apart for the next six months. When Sigmond received an overseas assignment at the Yokota Base in Japan, Louise applied for a transfer and soon joined her husband. For the next two years, Louise worked as a staff nurse in the base clinic while Sigmond flew with a strategic air command unit over Korea. In 1955, Sigmond's unit rotated back to the United States, and he was assigned to a post in Washington, DC. When Louise arrived four months later, she learned that her husband had suffered a disassociation reaction, which later developed into a chronic mental illness. The next few years were ones of struggle and turmoil for Louise. She worked part time while trying to balance caring for her husband and providing support to her brother, Kenneth, and his family during his illness. Louise finally came to the realization that, for her own mental health, she must proceed with a divorce, a decision that caused her considerable pain and anguish. The divorce, followed by her brother's death, left Louise feeling empty and lonely.

CLINICAL CENTER, NATIONAL INSTITUTES OF HEALTH

For financial reasons, Louise had to return to work full time. In 1958, Louise applied for a job at the Clinical Center at the National Institutes of Health (NIH) and was assigned to a cancer unit. At the time, she knew very little about caring for patients with cancer. She recalled that, although she was innocent as to what was in store for her, she was eager for a challenge and an opportunity to learn about what was new and experimental in cancer treatments. This was the beginning of Louise's career in cancer nursing that, for the next 25 years, would place her on the front lines of new and innovative programs and services for improving care to patients with cancer.

During Louise's orientation, she learned that her daily assignments would involve giving care to patients with metastatic breast disease following hypophysectomy or patients with carcinoma who were on clinical trials with new chemotherapy agents. She remembered the next two years at NIH as being some of the most satisfying as well as the most frustrating times of her nursing career. Pain control was very poor in those days. Nurses gave pain medications every four hours and never sooner, regardless of how much pain the patient was experiencing. Another difficulty was that the patients' cancer diagnosis or prognosis was not readily discussed, despite the fact that they knew they had cancer. On the other hand, because patients usually had long hospitalizations, staff nurses often established meaningful relationships with them and their family members. These connections gave purpose and a sense of accomplishment to the daily routines of care. The down side of these friendships was the intense feeling of loss that nurses experienced during a patient's death.

While a staff nurse, Louise had a chance meeting with a colleague from Pittsburgh, Agnus Campbell, who was working at the nearby naval hospital. Once again, Agnus convinced Louise to continue her education. Taking a two-year leave from the hospital and with financial aid provided by a federal training program, Louise entered Catholic University of America, and, in 1962, earned a master's degree in nursing. Her thesis examined the job satisfaction of staff nurses in a general hospital setting. Ninety-eight staff nurses completed the Science Research Associate Employee Inventory, which Louise used as data in determining if specific job factors had more influence on job satisfaction than others (Lunceford, 1962).

Upon returning to the Clinical Center, Louise requested a head nursing position. For the next 11 years, she managed the cancer care, which was provided by nurses, on two different units. One of these units was considered among the hardest to manage because of patient acuity and the emotional and physical stress. Patients ranged in age from 10 years old to adults and included adolescents with acute leukemia as well as adults with a variety of malignancies. Many of the patients were in the terminal phase of their disease and had come to the Clinical Center for clinical trials as a last effort to add days to their lives. The medical treatment orientation of the unit was incongruent with the frequent outcome of death. The dichotomy caused considerable emotional turmoil in the staff nurses, and they looked to Louise for support and understanding. Louise also recalled nurses mixing chemotherapy without having any knowledge of the hazards of handling toxic drugs. Because patients were participating in phase II trials, they sometimes received experimental drugs at dosing levels that led to septic shock, an emergency that required nurses to respond quickly. Louise organized a crash cart of emergency supplies that proved effective in providing the necessary equipment for an orderly and efficient treatment.

Creating a "milieu management" program for the more than 20 adolescents admitted to the leukemia service was a unique approach to caring for these teenagers. This program that Louise developed and implemented was based on the philosophy that patients are helped more when they are able to talk about their fears and anxieties. The "milieu management" environment promoted an understanding of adolescents as people. The goal was the freeing of anxiety in as many areas as possible to enable the patients to function more productively (Vernick & Lunceford, 1967).

A new technique of reverse isolation, the Life Island, was introduced at the Clinical Center in 1964. It called for a plan of nursing care that maintained a sterile environment for patients with extremely low resistance to infection (Lunceford, 1966). When two Life Island isolators were installed on the unit, Louise prepared the nurses to give special care to patients whose only hope

Nurses were skeptical when the Chemotherapy Service of the National Cancer Institute adopted a policy of honestly answering adolescents' questions about leukemia and death. But, they learned that answers brought more comfort to the children than evasions. Another policy with a difference is the provision of as much normal activity as possible for these youngsters.

VERNICK & LUNCEFORD, 1967, P. 559

JANET LOUISE MCKENZIE LUNCEFORD

for prolonged survival was to undergo intense chemotherapy. The Life Island consisted of a standard hospital bed surrounded by a plastic barrier to keep out environmental microorganisms. Long sleeves with rubber gloves were seamed into the plastic casing so that someone outside of the encasement could work within the protected area. A console at the foot of the bed was composed of a filter for air, two ultraviolet light locks for passing items into and out of the protected area, and a control panel to operate the unit. Patients undergoing intensive chemotherapy often remained in the Life Island for as long as three weeks. Nursing care was complex and time-consuming and required meticulous skills. Usually, nurses were assigned to only one patient for an entire shift. The quality of the patient's care depended primarily on the nurse's ability to plan and anticipate the needs of the patient.

In 1969, Laminar Air Flow Rooms replaced Life Island isolators. The goal for using these rooms was to provide a form of reverse isolation in which a patient could live in a fairly normal fashion for an extended period of time while receiving intensive IV chemotherapy (Lunceford, 1968). The Laminar Air Flow Room was a room within a room that had a horizontal air-flow pattern. Normal air passed through a prefilter and a bank of particulate air filters before entering the room. Preparation of the patient began five days before entry and required a prescribed medical protocol of bathing, cleansing, and teaching patients about the room. Louise described the vital role that nurses had in creating a normal living situation for the patient while simultaneously supporting medical efforts. Nurses had to enforce methodical control, design a sense of order, and establish routines that fostered a sense of security for the patient.

Even though Louise loved the patient contact, being responsible for the daily management of this unit plus studying patients with acute leukemia took its toll on her. She recognized the need for change and was granted a transfer to the Education and

BELOW
Laminar Air Flow Room

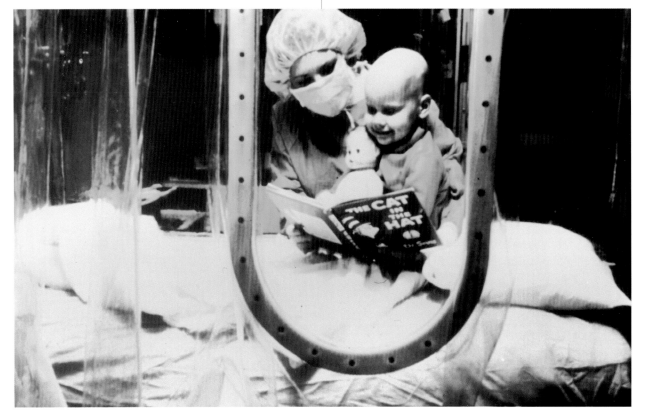

Training Unit of the Nursing Department at the Clinical Center. During the next four years, Louise worked on a variety of projects, including

- Coordinator and liaison for the Nursing Department's NIH Stride Nursing Program with Marymount Junior College in Virginia
- Development and implementation of a "Blood Administration Course"
- Participation in the Clinical Center's "Health-Care Workers Positive for Hepatitis B Surface Antigen" study
- Development and implementation of a work-study program in cancer nursing.

Louise identified the last project as the highlight of her time in the education department because the project reconnected her with cancer nursing. She looked forward to each summer when she supervised 20 senior baccalaureate students who came to the NIH campus to work at the Clinical Center. Several of the student nurses went on to become clinical cancer nursing experts. The American Cancer Society (ACS) cosponsored the work-study program, which meant that Louise also had the pleasure of working alongside Virginia Barckley.

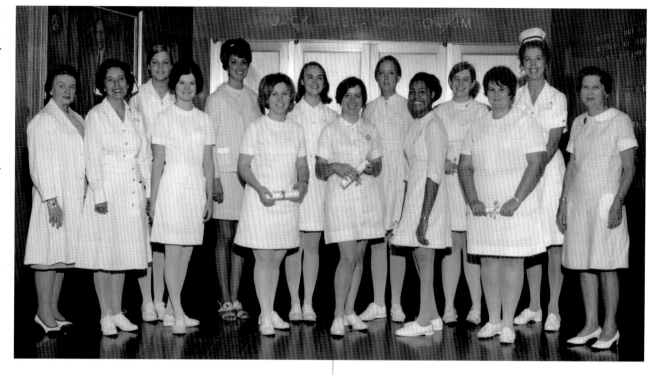

DIVISION OF CANCER CONTROL AND REHABILITATION, NATIONAL CANCER CENTER

When Louise learned that there was an opportunity to move from the Clinical Center to the Division of Cancer Control and Rehabilitation, she applied for the position, and in 1975, she became Program Director for Oncology Nursing. This position included being project officer for 15 continuing-education programs in cancer nursing, three enterostomal training programs, and one comprehensive rehabilitation program developed and implemented by oncology nurse coordinators.

Louise's travels across the country put her in touch with many of the leaders in oncology nursing, such as Jo Craytor at the University of Rochester Cancer Center in New York, Renilda

JANET LOUISE MCKENZIE LUNCEFORD

The hospice concept has begun a revolution in our American health care system and in the values of American people regarding terminal illness and care of the dying. Even studies and programs to improve long-term care of chronically ill and elderly patients have come to the forefront of national attention due to the emphasis on pain control and humane care of the patient and family experiencing terminal illness.

ABDELLAH, HARPER, & LUNCEFORD, 1982, P. 1

Hilkemeyer at the University of Texas M.D. Anderson Cancer Center, and Luana Lamkin at Queens Medical Center in Hawaii. Some of the three-year continuing-education programs were held in community hospitals, while others were awarded to universities. Louise was impressed with the instructors' eagerness and creativity in providing a quality learning experience for the nurses, with the amount of information being taught in the cancer courses, and with the enthusiasm that attendees had for learning about cancer care. In particular, Louise cited a community-based program in Waterbury, CT, which was directed by Charlotte Wright, as being one of the most successful. Charlotte strove to provide cancer education to all members of the care team, including the clergy. During the three years of the project, more than 5,000 people attended the oncology courses. Joan Piemme at Georgetown University directed a unique summer program for instructors and also found a way to hold continuing-education classes along with course work for undergraduate students.

In 1976, Dr. Diane Fink appointed Louise as Acting Chief of the Treatment, Rehabilitation, and Continuing Care branch. Louise recognized that this was not the best position, as it took her out of the role of nursing and placed her in an administrative role that included more meetings than she cares to remember. Her responsibilities included supervision of health professionals who directed and monitored contracts and grants, program administration of grants related to oncology nursing and clinical care of patients with cancer, and supervision of support personnel.

In 1980, Louise was appointed Program Director for Oncology Nursing, a position much more to her liking. She was responsible for developing and directing a post-master's fellowship contact program in oncology nursing. The program, intended for faculty members, was implemented at the University of Alabama and San Jose State University in California. Trainees were given an annual stipend of $10,000 along with their tuition. Course work was combined with time in the clinical setting. Nursing as a whole benefited from having this advanced-study opportunity. For example, Jane Fernsler, one of the nurse trainees, went on to establish a master's program in cancer nursing at the University of Delaware after completing the doctoral program.

Hospice care was beginning to evolve in this country. Louise, along with Faye Abdellah and Bernice Harper, two other nurse leaders at the federal level, prepared the government document on hospice care under the auspices of the Health Care Financing Administration. This government report, *Report on Hospice Care in the United States* (1982), provided a frame of reference for caregivers in improving their services to patients and family members. During the same time, under Louise's guidance, the National Cancer Institute (NCI) launched the Hospice Demonstration Project, which funded the development of three freestanding hospices: Hillhaven Foundation in Tucson, AZ, Kaiser-Permanente Medical Care Program, Los Angeles, CA, and Riverside Hospital in Boonton

Township, NJ. These hospices were to be modeled after the free-standing St. Christopher's Hospice in London in the belief that the freestanding hospice was the optimal milieu for providing care for terminally ill patients with cancer (Buck et al., 1985).

In addition to her work responsibilities, Louise offered her professional services and skills to several related organizations. She was a member of the ACS National Committee on Service and Rehabilitation from 1974–1980. She served as co-chairperson of the National Nursing Advisory Committee of ACS and, while in this role, helped to organize the 1977 ACS Conference on Cancer Nursing and the Second National Conference on Human Values and Cancer. In 1977, Louise was invited to become a member of the advisory board of the International Association for Enterstomal Therapy. She also was involved with the Leukemia Society of America, where she served as a trustee and chairperson of the Patient Aid Committee from 1973–1985. During this time, Barbara Bush became the honorary chairperson of the Leukemia Society. Louise had the distinct pleasure of meeting Mrs. Bush at a reception held in the home of the then Vice President George Bush.

ABOVE
Leukemia Society of America Reception
Louise Lunceford (right) with
Barbara Bush (left)

RETIREMENT

Louise retired from NIH in 1985 and, in that same year, moved from the Washington, DC area to San Diego, CA. She chose this location mainly to enjoy the sun and warmth of southern California. Louise decided to "drop out" of nursing when she retired but still maintains an interest in cancer nursing from a distance. For several years, Louise volunteered with the American Red Cross and helped families in crisis. She currently works one morning a week tutoring a girl in elementary school as part of the Seniors Helping Our Kids program. Louise takes frequent trips East to visit the families of her niece and nephew as well as her aunt who lives in Ohio.

At home, she keeps busy with her many social commitments, including involvement in the local art museum, theater, and music. The proliferation of computers has challenged Louise to learn new skills, especially the e-mail feature, as a way to connect with family and friends. Her small garden area around her condominium gives evidence of her love for gardening. Louise obviously has made a fulfilling and enjoyable transition into retirement.

JANET LOUISE MCKENZIE LUNCEFORD

SUMMARY

Louise Lunceford has had a very interesting and fulfilling career in cancer nursing that spanned many years. She began her career in cancer nursing at a time when new and innovative cancer treatment protocols called for highly skilled and compassionate nurses. Within the timeframe that she worked at the Clinical Center at NIH and with the Treatment, Rehabilitation, and Continuing Care branch of NCI, cancer shifted from being viewed as a disease you died from to being a chronic illness that you lived with. Louise's contributions to cancer nursing are reflective of this change in approach to cancer treatment and care. In reflecting on her own career, Louise had this to say when asked what of her life's work was most satisfying.

On a personal level, I am most pleased with the nursing care that I was able to deliver when working on the cancer unit. Those were poignant times but also were the most satisfying for me. I treasure those years and am proud of my role with the Life Island isolator and the Laminar Flow Room.

REFERENCES

Abdellah, F., Harper, B., & Lunceford, J.L. (1982). *Report on hospice care in the United States*. Washington, DC: U.S. Department of Health and Human Services—Health Care Financing Administration.

Buck, G., Cummings, M., Curran, B., Gotsch, A., Lunceford, J.L., Meudell, B., Muenz, L., Barofsky, I., & Grower, R. (1985). Hospice: A descriptive analysis of three programs. *Journal of Psychosocial Oncology, 3*(2), 83–96.

Lunceford, J.L. (1962). *Job satisfaction among selected general staff nurses in one general hospital*. Unpublished master's dissertation, School of Nursing, Catholic University of America, Washington, DC.

Lunceford, J.L. (1966). *Nursing care of patients in a Life Island isolator. Exploring progress in medical-surgical nursing practice*. New York: American Nurses Association.

Lunceford, J.L. (1968). Nursing care of patients in the laminar air flow room. In Nursing Department at National Institutes of Health (Ed.), *Nursing care of patients in the Laminar Flow Room: A nursing clinical conference* (p. 1). Bethesda, MD: National Institute of Health.

Oncology Nursing Society. (1987). *Those were the hard days* [Videotape]. (Available from the Oncology Nursing Society, 501 Holiday Drive, Pittsburgh, PA 15220)

Vernick, J., & Lunceford, J.L. (1967). Milieu design for adolescents with leukemia. *American Journal of Nursing, 67*, 559–561.

Lunceford, Janet Louise, interview by Judith Johnson, January 2000.

SELECTED WRITINGS
MILIEU DESIGN FOR ADOLESCENTS WITH LEUKEMIA (1967)

Nurses were skeptical when the Chemotherapy Service of the National Cancer Institute adopted a policy of honestly answering adolescents' questions about leukemia and death. But, they learned that answers brought more comfort to the children than evasions. Another policy with a difference is the provision of as much normal activity as possible for these youngsters.

Some persons might view a cancer nursing unit as one in which an atmosphere of dread and fear prevail. This atmosphere does not surround our twenty or more adolescent patients over a period of a year with leukemia on the Chemotherapy Service of the National Cancer Institute. For these children with all the normal adjustment problems of teenagers, the problems of adjusting to a hospital, and anxiety about impending death, we established an environment in which these adolescents could feel they were understood as persons. Our program, milieu management, is similar to those developed in residential treatment of emotionally disturbed children.

Our program is based on the philosophy that the patient is helped more by being able to talk about his fears and anxieties and problems—including the possibility of death—than by dealing with these problems alone.

The more a patient knows about his own condition and progress and those of his friends and other patients on the floor, the less anxious he becomes. Of course, all anxiety is not dissipated. But, our goal is the freeing of anxiety in as many areas as possible to enable the patients to function more productively.

The oft-used maxim, "treatment of the whole patient," is an actuality and not a fantasy.

Helping Patients Talk

To free a patient to talk about himself, his friends, and death, staff members must understand the serious predicament of the patient. This is crucial. The best way to communicate this understanding is to answer questions truthfully.

JANET LOUISE MCKENZIE LUNCEFORD

However, we recognize that all nurses cannot agree to or feel free to discuss such matters. Particularly at the outset of our program, there was much resistance. The general attitude expressed verbally and non-verbally was: The less these problems are discussed, the less upset the children will be. Also, some nurses thought milieu management would cost them time needed for physical care of patients.

Nurses also realized that the "extra" work was something that they could accomplish during such routine activities as giving medication and taking temperatures. As some staff members exhibited willingness to talk, patients were able to communicate more readily on a meaningful level.

It also needs to be pointed out that there were those on the nursing staff who were unable to involve themselves in such an emotional area, and in the final analysis, each person has to resolve such problems in the manner best suited to his own intellectual and emotional adjustment.

Note. From "Milieu Design for Adolescents With Leukemia," by J. Vernick and J.L. Lunceford, 1967, *American Journal of Nursing, 67*, pp. 559–561. Copyright 1967 by Lippincott Williams & Wilkins. Excerpted with permission.

NURSING CARE OF PATIENTS IN A LIFE ISLAND ISOLATOR (1965)

A new technique of reverse isolation—the Life Island—called for a new plan of nursing care to maintain a sterile environment for the patient undergoing cancer chemotherapy. This paper describes the Life Island system used by the Cancer Nursing Service of the National Institutes of Health Clinical Center, Bethesda, MD. The author is Head Nurse of the Cancer Nursing Service.

In recent months, the staff of the Cancer Nursing Service of the National Institutes of Health Clinical Center has worked with a relatively new system of reverse isolation—the Life Island. This is a protective technique designed for patients who are especially vulnerable to severe infection.

It is for this reason that the Life Island is utilized to protect the patient by giving him a bacteriologically controlled environment, as germ-free as man and science can provide. The system, of course, is set up in accordance with the medical criteria established for its use. The intensive cancer chemotherapy administered at the National Cancer Institute requires as sterile an environment as it is possible to create.

The Life Island isolator system used by the Cancer Institute consists of two major parts: the plastic enclosure and the console.

A flexible clear plastic enclosure surrounds a standard hospital-sized bed. Arm-length plastic sleeves, with rubber gloves, are fitted into the side walls of the tent. It is through these gloves that the patient receives care.

The tent is like a bubble, constructed in accordion-like fashion and supported on an overhead track. This design makes it possible for the nurse to move with relative ease when caring for the patient. It also permits access to the entire patient area inside the enclosure.

To prepare and orient the patient for the Life Island, the staff employs a team approach. First, the physician talks to the patient and his family about the proposed therapy and what he hopes to achieve by it. He assures himself that the patient wants this type of therapy, then arranges a conference for the patient and his family with the nurse supervisor of the project, the patient's physician, the dietitian, the medical social worker, and the hospital chaplain. All questions raised by the patient and his family are answered. Finally, the patient visits the Life Island itself and sees how it functions.

The nurse is responsible for maintaining the sterility of the patient's environment. Her ability to do so is reflected in bacteriology reports based on a continuous daily sample taken of the air that circulates inside the enclosure. If organisms other than those emanating from the patient himself were found on the air culture plates, it would indicate a possible break in sterile technique by the nurse; a break in the physical barrier, such as a large tear in the plastic enclosure; or the admission of non-sterile items into the Life Island.

PhisoHex is used in the patient's daily bath to assist in controlling the bacteriological count in the enclosure. In addition, the patient receives non-absorbable antibiotics which are bacteria-static. Oral pharyngeal sprays, Neomycin, Bactitracin and Nystatin are administered every two hours

JANET LOUISE MCKENZIE LUNCEFORD

while the patient is awake. The bacterial count in the intestinal tract is controlled by oral antibiotics which include Humatin, Sulfathalidine, Nystatin and Neomycin.

A nurse is assigned to the patient for each tour of duty. He is her sole responsibility. At the Clinical Center, this concentration of nursing care and observation is considered essential for the toxic, acutely ill patient. The quality of his care depends primarily on the nurse's ability to plan and anticipate, well in advance, the needs of the patient. This involves a knowledge of specific pieces of equipment needed, a maintenance of the sterility of all items, and the practice of good aseptic techniques.

It may be wondered how the patient can stand so much isolation and immobilization. The writer does not wish to minimize the importance of these restrictions, but when the reality of the patient's situation is analyzed, it does not seem so surprising that these patients have tolerated the experience very well. There are probably several reasons for this:

The Life Island offers the patient a real opportunity to prolong his life. Without treatment, his survival could be limited to weeks. Also, reverse isolation is a protective technique; therefore, the patient does not have the feeling of contamination as does the patient appropriately isolated with an infectious disease.

The life island permits the hospital staff, the patient's family and visitors to move freely around the room with no necessity to wear the customary isolation garments: gowns, gloves and mask.

Finally, since the nurse devotes all her time to caring for the patient in the Life Island, there is ample opportunity for a mutually satisfactory relationship to develop. Evidence that this has happened was supplied by our first patient who, after his sojourn in the Life Island, was asked, "What were the things that made the experience easier for you?"

He replied: "The nurses. Their constant presence was comforting."

TRIBUTES

As principal investigator at the University of Alabama School of Nursing, I traveled to Washington, DC, for the first of several meetings about the post-master's program in oncology nursing education. Louise served as the project officer for this innovative and unique NCI contact, which required that she facilitate collaboration between the University of Alabama School of Nursing and the San Jose State University School of Nursing. The focus of the project was the preparation of oncology nurse educators at the post-master's level. Not only were the schools at different ends of the United States, with geographic and cultural variability, but each faculty group had different levels of experience in graduate education and oncology nursing. Louise was a great coordinator and resource person for us as we developed curricula, instructional strategies, and evaluative processes that met both the project objectives and reflected our uniqueness. Her site visits always were eagerly anticipated not only because of the opportunity to share our progress with her and to obtain her insights and suggestions but also because she was a fun guest at dinner. I always will be grateful to her not only for teaching me the politics of federal grant funding and the value of interinstitutional collaboration but also the rewards that come to those in cancer nursing education.

Anne E. Belcher, RN, PhD, AOCN®, FAAN

Associate Professor
University of Maryland School of Nursing
Baltimore, MD

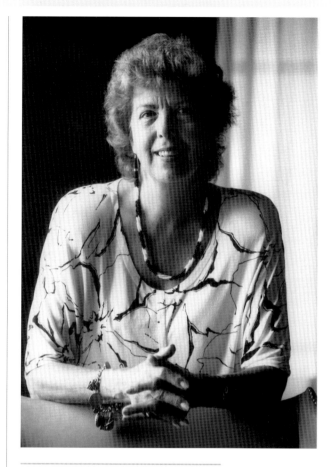

ABOVE
J. Louise Lunceford

An indelible memory that I have of Louise is her ready smile, her words of encouragement, and her "can do" philosophy to grantees in the community continuing-education programs. Long before collaborative efforts became the norm in nursing practice and education, Louise brought all of the grantees together on an annual basis to share ideas, successful innovations, and lessons learned.

As the principal investigator on one of these community continuing-education programs, I was able to design and implement curricula that were not feasible within the existing academic structure. The grant afforded Louise the opportunity to design the first clinical nursing elective in the School of Nursing at Georgetown University. For those of us who worked with Louise during this point in her career, we believed that her creativity made significant contributions to the advancement of the cancer nursing practice and education in the academic setting.

Joan A. Piemme, RN, MNEd, FAAN

Oncology and HIV Nursing Educator
Harpers Ferry, WV

Personal papers and effects of Janet Louise Lunceford are located in the archives at the National Office of the Oncology Nursing Society in Pittsburgh, PA.

EPILOGUE

In 12 short chapters, we have presented the biographies of a representative group of outstanding women who pioneered in cancer nursing practice, education, and research from the late 19th century through the early 1970s. We used multiple resources to gather the information from which we fashioned each individual's story, striving always to portray each subject as clearly as possible, without bias. To this end, we read and reread their writings and what has been written about them, poured over their memorabilia, interviewed selected colleagues of each, and conducted hours of in-person and telephone interviews with each of the featured women who are still living. The process was challenging and exhilarating. We felt privileged to share so much of their personal lives and grateful that these cancer nursing leaders were willing to have their personal recollections shared with our readers. Their stories are all different, yet common threads of influence and direction are woven from chapter to chapter, shaping their lives, their careers, and the direction of oncology nursing as it is practiced today in the 21st century.

Consider the role of science and medicine as it evolved in the 20th century. The very nature of science was, at best, haphazard in its evolution, sometimes producing progress in the absence of understanding. These cancer nursing pioneers began to tackle the vagueness of nursing practice and education, coaxing theory into a visible, manageable, and user-friendly format that would stimulate the current excellence in practice, education, and research. They challenged the status quo of the nurse's role, pushed for increased funding for oncology nursing education, and developed collegial relationships with members of the other oncology practice disciplines. Most of all, these early cancer nurses struggled to place the needs of patient and family first and foremost in cancer care and treatment.

The direction that our subjects' careers followed was heavily influenced by the social, economic, and political climate of the time. Rose Hawthorne Lathrop was drawn to the poorest of the poor in New York City, and her decision to dedicate her life to terminally ill patients with cancer was based upon her spiritual conviction and a deep social conscience.

Marriage, health, serious illness in family members, and personal choices led some of these cancer nursing pioneers to a new focus and, thus, onto their paths of achievement.

Florence Wald and Katherine Nelson began their professional lives in health-related but non-nursing careers. They, like Jeanne Quint Benoliel, Louise Lunceford, and Rosalie Peterson, personally were affected by wars that was inserted into the lives and social fabric of this nation. Changes in the philosophy of adult education, greater acceptance of college education for women, and the loosening of some of the barriers to women in academia were significant factors in the lives and careers of several of our subjects. Jeanne Quint Benoliel was a major force in breaking the barriers to nursing's participation in scientific research. Likewise, Jo Craytor pioneered in elevating nursing's role in the clinical setting to one of collaboration with medical colleagues, in spite of resistance from physicians and nurses alike. Doris Diller immersed herself in medical education to better serve as a patient advocate. Her close working relationship with the medical discipline led to her co-authorship of a surgical nursing textbook with a physician.

When reading these biographies, it becomes clear that the evolution of oncology as a distinct discipline and the establishment of major cancer centers, like Memorial Sloan-Kettering in New York City and M.D. Anderson in Houston, TX, also influenced the development of oncology nursing. Advances in science and technology meant that nurses were further challenged to meet the patients' needs. The leaders featured in this text saw the need for cancer nursing education and found the means to make this a reality. In doing so, they collaborated with government, academic, and voluntary organizations, bringing these diverse groups together for the common purpose of patient care and improved quality of life. The National Cancer Institute often was the funding source that underwrote these nurses' projects.

One of the more significant relationships that was forged in the evolution of cancer nursing was that between nurses and the American Cancer Society (ACS). Nurses have been instrumental in helping to carry out the mission of ACS; while at the same time, ACS has provided resources for the advancement of cancer nursing practice, education, and research. Many of the leaders featured in this text had ties to ACS throughout their professional lives

Recruitment, education, and retention of oncology nurses have been ongoing challenges. Episodic nursing shortages combined with negative public attitudes toward cancer led Norma Owens to the development of the Nurse Internship Program at New York University. Edith Wolf constantly was motivated by the need to recruit nurses for the demands of nursing care at the Memorial Hospital for Cancer and Allied Diseases. Virginia Barckley tackled the problem of nursing recruitment by collaborating with Renilda Hilkemeyer to bring students to major cancer centers for intensive clinical experience.

The evolution and history of oncology nursing does not end with this book. We deliberately have chosen to chronicle only some of the nurses whose work has preceded the founding of the Oncology Nursing Society in 1975. In fact, as we leave the task of documenting the continuing evolution of our specialty to a new generation, we stand in awe of the sheer number of oncology nurses, the depth of their knowledge, and the breadth of their contributions to patient care, professional education, and scientific inquiry. Survival, rehabilitation, and advocacy have taken on a whole new meaning. Consider the leap in knowledge of cell biology, genetics, carcinogenesis, holistic medicine and complementary therapies, pharmaceuticals, radiobiology, combined modality treatment, and the advantages of multidisciplinary care. We can say with great pride and deep respect that oncology nurses are among the leaders, pioneers, movers, and shakers in the burgeoning body of knowledge related to oncology science and care in the early 21st century. We hope that the *Courage, Compassion, and Curiosity* of oncology nursing leaders will continue to be documented, published, and shared with all.

JUDITH BOND JOHNSON
SUSAN B. BAIRD
LAURA J. HILDERELY